VOLUME

LIZ STILLWAGGON SWAN has a PhD in philosophy and is a certified yoga instructor. Her niche in the world is helping people exercise their brains and their bodies. Her recent publications in the emerging field of biosemiotics explore how we use our brains and bodies to make sense of the world. She is also a new mother and delights in watching her son practice happy baby pose.

SERIES EDITOR

FRITZ ALLHOFF is an associate professor in the philosophy department at Western Michigan University, as well as a senior research fellow at the Australian National University's Centre for Applied Philosophy and Public Ethics. In addition to editing the *Philosophy for Everyone series*, he is also the volume editor or co-editor for several titles, including *Wine & Philosophy* (Wiley-Blackwell, 2007), *Whiskey & Philosophy* (with Marcus P. Adams, Wiley, 2009), and *Food & Philosophy* (with Dave Monroe, Wiley-Blackwell, 2007). His academic research interests engage various facets of applied ethics, ethical theory, and the history and philosophy of science.

PHILOSOPHY FOR EVERYONE

Series editor: Fritz Allhoff

Not so much a subject matter, philosophy is a way of thinking. Thinking not just about the Big Questions, but about little ones too. This series invites everyone to ponder things they care about, big or small, significant, serious … or just curious.

Running & Philosophy:
A Marathon for the Mind
Edited by Michael W. Austin

Wine & Philosophy:
A Symposium on Thinking and Drinking
Edited by Fritz Allhoff

Food & Philosophy:
Eat, Think and Be Merry
Edited by Fritz Allhoff and Dave Monroe

Beer & Philosophy:
The Unexamined Beer Isn't Worth Drinking
Edited by Steven D. Hales

Whiskey & Philosophy:
A Small Batch of Spirited Ideas
Edited by Fritz Allhoff and Marcus P. Adams

College Sex – Philosophy for Everyone: Philosophers With Benefits
Edited by Michael Bruce and Robert M. Stewart

Cycling – Philosophy for Everyone:
A Philosophical Tour de Force
Edited by Jesús Ilundáin-Agurruza and Michael W. Austin

Climbing – Philosophy for Everyone:
Because It's There
Edited by Stephen E. Schmid

Hunting – Philosophy for Everyone:
In Search of the Wild Life
Edited by Nathan Kowalsky

Christmas – Philosophy for Everyone:
Better Than a Lump of Coal
Edited by Scott C. Lowe

Cannabis – Philosophy for Everyone:
What Were We Just Talking About?
Edited by Dale Jacquette

Porn – Philosophy for Everyone:
How to Think With Kink
Edited by Dave Monroe

Serial Killers – Philosophy for Everyone : Being and Killing
Edited by S. Waller

Dating – Philosophy for Everyone:
Flirting With Big Ideas
Edited by Kristie Miller and Marlene Clark

Gardening – Philosophy for Everyone:
Cultivating Wisdom
Edited by Dan O'Brien

Motherhood – Philosophy for Everyone: The Birth of Wisdom
Edited by Sheila Lintott

Fatherhood – Philosophy for Everyone: The Dao of Daddy
Edited by Lon S. Nease and Michael W. Austin

Coffee – Philosophy for Everyone:
Grounds for Debate
Edited by Scott F. Parker and Michael W. Austin

Fashion – Philosophy for Everyone:
Thinking with Style
Edited by Jessica Wolfendale and Jeanette Kennett

Yoga – Philosophy for Everyone:
Bending Mind and Body
Edited by Liz Stillwaggon Swan

Forthcoming books in the series:

Blues – Philosophy for Everyone:
Thinking Deep About Feeling Low
Edited by Abrol Fairweather and Jesse Steinberg

Sailing – Philosophy for Everyone:
A Place of Perpetual Undulation
Edited by Patrick Goold

Tattoos – Philosophy for Everyone:
I Ink, Therefore I Am
Edited by Rob Arp

Edited by Liz Stillwaggon Swan

YOGA
PHILOSOPHY FOR EVERYONE
Bending Mind and Body

Foreword by John Friend

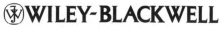
WILEY-BLACKWELL
A John Wiley & Sons, Ltd., Publication

This edition first published 2012
© 2012 John Wiley & Sons, Inc.

Wiley-Blackwell is an imprint of John Wiley & Sons, formed by the merger of
Wiley's global Scientific, Technical and Medical business with Blackwell Publishing.

Registered Office
John Wiley & Sons Ltd, The Atrium, Southern Gate, Chichester, West Sussex,
PO19 8SQ, UK

Editorial Offices
350 Main Street, Malden, MA 02148-5020, USA
9600 Garsington Road, Oxford, OX4 2DQ, UK
The Atrium, Southern Gate, Chichester, West Sussex, PO19 8SQ, UK

For details of our global editorial offices, for customer services, and for information
about how to apply for permission to reuse the copyright material in this book please
see our website at www.wiley.com/wiley-blackwell.

The right of Liz Stillwaggon Swan to be identified as the author of the editorial
material in this work has been asserted in accordance with the UK Copyright,
Designs and Patents Act 1988.

Library of Congress Cataloging-in-Publication Data
Yoga – philosophy for everyone : bending mind and body / edited by
Liz Stillwaggon Swan.
   p. cm. – (Philosophy for everyone)
  ISBN 978-0-470-65880-2 (pbk. : alk. paper)
1. Hatha yoga. 2. Yoga–Philosophy. I. Swan, Liz Stillwaggon, 1973–
  RA781.7.Y628 2012
  613.7′046–dc23
                            2011020594

A catalogue record for this book is available from the British Library.

This book is published in the following electronic formats: ePDFs 9781118121429;
Wiley Online Library 9781118121450; ePub 9781118121436; Mobi 9781118121443

Set in 10/12.5pt Plantin by SPi Publisher Services, Pondicherry, India
Printed in Malaysia by Ho Printing (M) Sdn Bhd

1   2012

For Freeman Jack Swan

CONTENTS

Foreword   ix
John Friend

Editor's Introduction   xiv
Liz Stillwaggon Swan

Acknowledgments   xxvi

PART 1   COMING INTO THE SPACE: WHAT IS YOGA?   1

1   How Yoga Won the West   3
Jennifer Munyer

2   Will I Find My Guru in India?   15
Kieran McManus

3   The Seeker: *How Yoga is Meeting Changing Western
Spiritual Needs*   24
David Robles

4   Men, Sports, and Yoga   36
Barbara Purcell and Andrew Shaffer

5   Standing on Your Head, Seeing Things Right Side Up   47
Steve Jacobson

PART 2   THE *ASANAS*: YOGA AND THE BODY   59

6   Help! My Philosophy Teacher Made Me Touch My Toes!   61
Ken Burak

7   Man a Machine, Man a Yogi: *Why Yoga's Critics will Come Around*   73
J. Neil Otte

8   Yoga for Women? *The Problem of Beautiful Bodies*   84
Luna Dolezal

9   The Feeling of Beauty: *A Yoga Project*   94
Nicole Dunas

10 Picturing Yoga: Yoga Journal *and the Perfect Form*   106
Debra Merskin

PART 3   *PRANA:* YOGA'S VITAL ENERGY   117

11 My Guidance Counselor Always Said I'd be a Great Yoga Student   119
Eric Swan

12 Balance in Yoga and Aristotle   129
Leigh Duffy

13 Healing the Western Mind through Yoga   139
Abby Thompson

14 The Path to Happiness Begins with a Journey Inside   149
Jim Berti

PART 4   *YAMAS* AND *NIYAMAS:* ETHICS AND YOGA   159

15 Get Out of My Way! I'm Late for Yoga!   161
Jeff Logan

16 Yoga Off the Mat   166
Julinna Oxley

17 Becoming-Frog: *Yoga as Environmentalism*   178
Megan M. Burke

18 Yoga and Ethics: *The Importance of Practice*   187
Paul Ulhas MacNeill

19 Why are You Standing on my Yoga Mat?!   200
Heather Salazar

Notes on Contributors   212

FOREWORD

Today, millions around the world regularly practice yoga. Yet many are unaware of the historical foundations of yoga and its underlying philosophies. Yoga: Philosophy for Everyone is an intellectually stimulating collection of nineteen thought-provoking essays that discuss yoga practice as it applies to twenty-first-century mainstream society. It presents some of the key ideas of the traditional lineages of yoga philosophy, while relating them to Western thought and culture through the writings of philosophers such as Aristotle and Descartes. Aptly titled, it covers a broad survey of topics, including life philosophy and diet, that are of great interest to both Western and Eastern cultures. This book, as its title implies and like yoga itself, is appropriate for everyone – from the beginner to the advanced practitioner and scholar.

For thousands of years in India, 'yoga' referred to both a state of cosmic consciousness and the disciplined practice that led the yogi into that state of ultimate spiritual union. The philosophy of yoga has endured over centuries because it has proven to be amazingly effective at explaining how to live in accordance with nature for greater health, happiness, and wisdom. Within the last 150 years the world has become increasingly exposed to the fundamental philosophical ideas of this life-enhancing practice. Today yoga philosophy is having profound influence in the areas of modern medicine, culture, interpersonal relationships, business, ethics, sports, and even cutting-edge scientific technology. So, with its increasing importance in the world today as an effective means for cultivating happiness and wisdom, everyone can benefit by understanding the basics of yoga philosophy.

The most common form of yoga practiced today worldwide is Hatha yoga, which focuses primarily on physical postures and breathing exercises. The cultural popularity of Hatha yoga has grown tremendously over the last twenty years, such that today yoga is practiced by tens of millions of people around the world. Not long ago the popular image of a yogi was a skinny man in a contorted, pretzel-like position disengaged from the mainstream of society. In stark contrast, the twenty-first-century image of a yoga practitioner is a young, fit, educated woman in her twenties or thirties. Although yoga is now so much more mainstream than at any other time in history, it is still not widely practiced by men, or non-white or overweight people.

Over the centuries, yoga practice has encompassed meditation, chanting, ritualistic Hindu worship ceremonies, the study of ancient scripture, the performance of intensely austere physical postures, and advanced breathing practices, all of which have not been easily integrated into our modern, high-speed, technological lives. Consequently, ancient yoga practices have been progressively modified for modern times. In just the last century, while underlying yoga philosophy has remained consistent, the modern yoga practice has morphed its outer form to the point that it hardly resembles its ancient, original form. It is important to note that both the philosophy and practice of yoga have always been living and breathing, never static. So, for practitioners today to continue to adapt the practice to fit into the world today is, in fact, very much in alignment with the entire history of yoga. The key to this evolution is to ensure that we are moving forward in innovative ways that are still rooted in the traditional fundamentals.

In the past, Hatha yoga poses were never performed separately from their spiritual context of yoga philosophy, including yogic ethics. However, since yoga began to be regularly broadcast on American television fifty years ago, it has become increasingly tied in the West to physical fitness and therapy, stress reduction, and personal empowerment, while becoming progressively disconnected from its Hindu roots and much of its essential philosophical foundations. It is common today for 'yoga' to be taught at health clubs and other venues around the world simply as a physical workout without any allusion to its ancient spiritual philosophy. Yoga has become so popular that in the last twenty years it has grown from a multi-million-dollar industry to a worldwide industry worth billions.

Today there are many styles or schools of Hatha yoga, several of which have been formed since only the 1970s in the United States. The main yoga schools include Iyengar, Bikram, Ashtanga Vinyasa, Kripalu, Baptiste,

JOHN FRIEND

Forrest, Jivamukti, Core Power, Yin, Pure, and Anusara yoga. Some of these schools have trademarked their brands, franchised their yoga studio businesses, and copyrighted their postural sequences. Currently, the various yoga schools do not agree on a universal definition of the practice of yoga. Each school ascribes to varying viewpoints on different aspects of yoga philosophy, including metaphysics, the structure of consciousness, and cosmology.

While different yoga schools have varied definitions of the yogic state and the necessary disciplined practice to achieve that state, a basic definition of yoga has stood the test of time. From the earliest mentions in Sanskrit texts, the word 'yoga' represented a state of individual awareness united with a universal presence. The Sanskrit root of the word is '*yuj*,' which means to unite, marry, yoke, or to turn two into one. In all of the practices of yoga throughout history there has always been a vision of becoming absorbed into supreme consciousness, the essence of reality and being. Yoga is an age-old spiritual practice that uses various mind–body techniques to unite individual consciousness – the soul – with its most essential source – supreme spirit. This ultimate union is characterized by a dissolving of the awareness of individual distinction and separateness until there is an experience of universality and boundlessness of consciousness.

Although all yoga schools will agree that 'yoga' fundamentally means 'union with the supreme,' there are significant differences in general yoga philosophy among the Hatha yoga schools worldwide. The key reason for this is that historically there are at least three different ancient philosophical systems that inform the modern yoga student: Classical Yoga, Vedanta, and Tantra.

In a Classical Yoga viewpoint, originally delineated by Patañjali in his *Yoga Sutras*, written sometime between 100 BCE and 500 CE, yoga means a separation of *purusha* (spirit) from its entangled identity with *prakriti* (matter). The goal of Classical Yoga is *kaivalya*, which means to 'isolate' spiritual consciousness from the lower-grade energy field, its mind–body. In Classical Yoga, matter includes the energetic field of thoughts, emotions, and the physical body, while above this vibratory matrix of mind–body is *purusha*, or pure being (spirit). Thus, the intention of Classical Yoga is to free or separate *purusha* from *prakriti* in order to abide in one's pure being, isolated and apart from any suffering.

In Vedantic yogic philosophy, yoga is a path toward recognition that a pure level of consciousness (spirit) is always present in everyone and all things in the material realm. Consciousness is cloaked by a power called *maya*, an illusion-causing creative force that is independent of the ground of pure consciousness. In Vedanta philosophy, yoga is defined as a path of awakening that takes place as the reality-distorting power of *maya* is neutralized through a yogi's practices. Once *maya*'s power is neutralized, the idea is that the grand unity of being is unveiled in the consciousness of the practitioner. When one remembers their true nature as oneness, there is direct experience of yoga. In this specific philosophical viewpoint, the nature of being is synonymous with *ananda*, the highest bliss and joy imaginable, so, in Vedanta, yoga is ultimately a state of realization with one's own true, blissful nature, which is not separate from the supreme.

Traditional, non-dual Tantric philosophy defines 'yoga' as a state of union with the very essence of *Shiva-Shakti*, or supreme consciousness and its creative power. This is the absolute level of reality that infinitely vibrates with pure auspiciousness, bliss, self-luminous awareness, freedom, and fullness of being. In contrast to Classical Yoga, Tantra philosophy sees both *purusha* and *prakriti* as having the same essence of Shiva-Shakti; since everything is supreme and pure consciousness at its essence, there is no need for isolation and separation. In contrast to Vedanta, Tantra sees *maya* not as an illusion but rather as the differentiating power of consciousness itself; a playful kind of power that allows individual souls to experience a variety of divine creative expressions of supreme consciousness.

The yogic practices within Tantra encompass a wide variety of subtle energy control, from the chanting of mantras, magickal (i.e., transforming matter by use of Shakti, as opposed to 'magic,' which refers to stage magic or sleight of hand) sounds and words, to breath-control and the use of *yantras* and *mandalas* (magickal diagrams). All Tantric yoga practices include the use of sophisticated techniques to affect subtle energy within the mind–body and the surrounding environment. In general, Tantric schools either seek power as the highest goal or delight as the pinnacle of *sadhana* (spiritual practice). Knowledge is both power and bliss in Tantra, so expansion of knowledge and awareness is a key endeavor. The goals of these energy-control techniques differ between specific Tantric schools, and range from life extension to increasing worldly power to experiencing the ultimate blissful freedom of the soul while embodied. All Hatha yoga practices derive from Tantric philosophy, in which the body and mind are considered different frequencies of the one supreme divine energy that fills everything in the universe.

Over the centuries, the yoga philosophies of Classical Yoga, Vedanta, and Tantra have remained consistent. However, modern yoga has embraced different elements of each of these philosophies, so there is not

JOHN FRIEND

one, consistent philosophical foundation for all Hatha yoga practices today. Certainly, one agreed-upon belief in all yoga schools is that yoga is a disciplined practice in which one lives the principles of one's philosophy instead of just intellectually knowing about them. There is knowledge gained indirectly from studying the yoga philosophy texts, and there is also the knowledge directly gained from deeply experiencing a moment of living that philosophy. It is commonly agreed that the direct knowledge gained from applying the philosophy in daily living, in contrast to just thinking or talking about it, is a higher or more effective path.

The higher knowledge of all yoga philosophical schools arises from the direct experience of one's spiritual essence through the various tried-and-true paths of yoga. The one truth central in the broad spectrum of all yoga philosophy is that the essence of being is free. Whether self, *purusha*, soul, or *atman*, whatever you want to call the individualized essence of the universal spirit is ultimately free in its true nature. Pure being is free from the suffering associated with the misidentification of itself with the changing materialistic world of embodiment. It is free from the illusionary veil that distorts our vision to see difference in a boundless field of unity. The self is pure awareness, unlimited consciousness eternally existing in a state of ultimate freedom.

Since that is the true nature at the core of our being, everyone seeks that experience when it is cloaked within our relative, embodied existence. Consequently, everyone who comes to yoga is ultimately seeking freedom. Freedom from suffering and the freedom to be happy are the root intentions behind anyone's choice to begin a yoga practice. At this critical time in Earth's history – environmentally, economically, politically, and culturally – may everyone gain deep insight from the basic knowledge of yoga philosophy to live in ways that bring more harmony, happiness, and love, and the joy of freedom to the world.

May *Yoga: Philosophy for Everyone* be a support and inspiration to all levels of yoga students. May all the ideas presented in this book help to deepen our embodiment of yogic ethical wisdom and compassion during these critical times on the Earth.

EDITOR'S INTRODUCTION

A few years ago, when I told a friend I was thinking about doing yoga teacher training he said, 'Wow. That's really serious. You're going to have to give up coffee and alcohol.' I was dumbfounded. What did he mean? What did drinking coffee, or anything else for that matter, have to do with yoga? Furthermore, if becoming a yoga teacher meant that I *would* have to find a way to squelch my love of coffee (and red wine), then my bright future as a yogini was in serious trouble. But more to the point, I had already been practicing yoga for a few years by then, and living a healthy lifestyle, without restricting myself in any sort of regimented or prescribed way. Having been raised Catholic, I was familiar with the idea of ritualistically giving up certain things as part of a tradition (e.g., giving up chocolate during Lent, the forty-day period leading up to Easter Sunday) but such practices didn't resonate with me as an adult. As an independent thinker and philosopher, the adoption of particular practices, such as avoiding certain substances, has to make sense to me for reasons I've arrived at myself. And, for me, yoga was not a religion, or even a spiritual practice. It was, and is, something that I love to do because of how it makes me feel.

In reading the nineteen essays in this book, you'll discover that yoga is something different to each person. There is no universal definition of yoga that applies to all yoga traditions or to all people who practice yoga. And certainly, yoga feels different to each one of us who experiences it. For me, moving and breathing through a series of yoga poses makes me feel grounded, calm, and content. And, as you might imagine, the more I generate such feelings through my yoga practice, the more I find myself feeling grounded, calm, and content in other parts of my day and my life. A favorite yoga teacher of mine who has written for this book, Jeff Logan, spoke in class one day about the powerful effect that simply imagining yourself in a calming yoga pose can have. For example, one pose I enjoy practicing is triangle pose, because I feel both grounded and expansive in this pose. And, because the body has memory, when I'm in a stressful situation such as going into a job interview, the act of recalling myself in triangle pose elicits in me the same positive feelings I experience when I'm actually in the pose – enabling me to enter the interview with a smile and sense of calm confidence.

You may be thinking that, as good as all this sounds, it doesn't seem *spiritual*, and that's what you thought yoga was all about. To understand why I don't think of yoga as a spiritual practice, I need to explain a bit about where I'm coming from philosophically. In college, when I was introduced to the philosophy of René Descartes – who, in the early seventeenth century, declared that minds (or 'spirits') and bodies were two different kinds of things in the world – I knew that he was wrong. I've spent a lot of time – probably too much time – explaining in philosophy papers exactly why I think he was wrong.

I offer here the nutshell version of my argument: There is no such thing as 'a mind' per se; rather, the term 'mind' acts as a conceptual placeholder for a whole host of abilities that we and some other animals are able to do with our brains and bodies working in concert, such as communicate, show affection, imagine, learn, play, and so on. An important source of inspiration for my early philosophical musings was the progressively minded contemporary of Descartes, Baruch Spinoza, who believed that the mental and the physical were two manifestations of a single, underlying reality. Consistent with this insight is the notion that all living organisms have a host of abilities uniquely attuned to their particular environments, which in some cases – for example, the human case – we're inclined to conceptualize as 'having a mind.'

When I began my yoga teacher training several months after having that curious conversation with my friend, I was surprised to find how much emphasis was placed on the idea that yoga means 'union' – commonly explained as the union between mind and body. I'd never believed that mind and body were separate in the first place, and these 'insights' seemed a curious, regressive step backward from Western philosophy's focus, over the past 400 years, on moving past Descartes' mind–body dualism. After a few lectures on how yoga helps one to integrate or unite mind and body, I felt like exclaiming: But I am an integrated whole! In essence, mind–body integration is a non-issue when we recognize that humans are animals with interesting abilities, as are all creatures on Earth. If nothing else, my yoga training made me question the popular assumption that Eastern philosophy is somehow one-up on Western philosophy when it comes to understanding the relationship between mind and body. I don't believe this is the case.

Historically, both Eastern and Western philosophical traditions have made the mistake of assuming that humans are somehow special in the natural world, unique among animals – for example, because we alone have a mind, or a soul, or are bound for some sort of afterlife – and these assumptions have created some very messy systems of beliefs. But yoga doesn't have to be messy, philosophically speaking; essentially, if one doesn't believe that there is a spirit (or mind) that exists separately from the body, then one cannot genuinely understand yoga as a practice of unifying mind and body.

But the fact remains that 'yoga' means union. Of what, then, is yoga a practice of 'uniting'? Megan Burke, who has written an essay for this book, offers an alternative interpretation of yogic union, beautiful in its simplicity, as one of uniting self with nature. She explains how yoga helps us to become more aware of the physical space around us, and in turn how this contextual awareness can be expanded off the mat and into the wider world of other living beings, and even to the natural world itself. Again, yoga is something different for each one of us, and, even without its being spiritual, yoga can be an amazingly powerful, transformative, and insightful practice.

Moreover, there may be advantages to *not* conceptualizing yoga as a spiritual practice. As a non-religious American born in the twentieth century, I feel comfortable introducing my yoga students to the physical benefits and relaxation techniques of yoga without making any references to the spiritual teachings of Hinduism in ancient India. When I teach a diverse group of yoga students at the local recreation center, I accept that some are there to have a spiritual experience while some are there to work on their balance, or because they've heard yoga can help lower their blood pressure. There are people who are drawn to yoga for the physical and psychological benefits it offers and are not seeking spiritual enlightenment because it just doesn't fit with their worldview. A point expressed compellingly in Julinna Oxley's essay in this book is that yoga is (or should be!) an inclusive practice, open and welcoming to all people with diverse backgrounds, some of whom consider it a spiritual pathway and some of whom do not.

There are some efforts in the yoga world today to garner some sort of recognition of yoga's ancient roots because, the argument goes, yoga as it is practiced today in the West is so far removed from its ancient origins in India. I believe these efforts are misguided. Almost everyone accepts that yoga began in India in ancient times, and I believe it is apparent that today's multi-billion-dollar yoga industry bears little resemblance to its ancestral past. To draw an analogy: We all know that Christmas day historically marks the birth of Jesus Christ in Bethlehem over 2000 years ago; but, for many who don't consider themselves Christians, Christmas is about spending time with family and friends, telling stories about Santa Claus and the elves, and drinking eggnog while decorating the Christmas tree. It would be unrealistic to insist in today's Western culture that everyone who celebrates Christmas must revere its historical origin in Bethlehem. Cultural practices evolve, and, although the yoga of today is a very different practice from that of long ago, this does not at all diminish the powerful movement that it is in today's world.

A sentiment that is also commonly heard from the yoga world is that yoga is 'not just exercise.' B. K. S. Iyengar explained this sentiment more eloquently when he said that practicing the yoga *asanas* (physical postures) without the study of yoga philosophy amounted to mere acrobatics. In other words, if your intention is simply to break a sweat and get a good workout, that can be satisfied by an aerobics class, or thirty minutes on the treadmill. It is true that yoga, as a physical practice, offers something more, with its focus on maintaining mindful breathing throughout the postures, no matter how challenging the pose being attempted may be. And yoga offers much more than that, with its rich history of yogic philosophy that covers everything related to being a good person and living a good life, for those who are eager for it.

However, at a time when in the United States roughly two thirds of all adults and one third of all children are obese or overweight – with the rest of the West not far behind – and with these rates rising sharply along with their attendant maladies such as diabetes and heart disease, it seems unwise to dismiss anything as 'mere exercise.' Not everyone will garner spiritual benefits from yoga, or even want to, but *everyone* can garner physical and psychological benefits from yoga. In fact, the essay in this book by my husband, Eric Swan, advocates for yoga being introduced to school-aged children as part of their personal and social development. To this I would add, their physical development too, since kids naturally take to yoga and find it fun. Bring on the acrobatics!

Yoga is well suited to help in the effort, currently being championed by First Lady Michelle Obama in the United States, to curb perilously rising rates of obesity in the West. First, there is a direct correlation between regular exercise and a healthy weight. As long as we use as much energy as we consume, we should maintain a healthy weight, and yoga is a very rewarding way of expending energy. But the same could be said for any form of exercise. What yoga has to offer nations of people facing major public health crises is a holistic, healthy, self-disciplined way of life, which includes healthy eating habits. One promise of yoga is that a well-disciplined body, which comes about over time through the practice of the yoga postures coupled with mindful breathing, can give rise to a well-disciplined mind. In other words, the more we learn to maintain our calm focus in challenging yoga practices, the more easily we find it to concentrate on demanding mental tasks and to stay focused and present in all intellectually challenging situations, including self-disciplined habits that go along with a healthy and nutritious lifestyle.

I had been studying Western analytic philosophy for many years when I first came to yoga, and thus had an easier time than some embodying the yogic principles of alignment, balance, depth, and precision in the postures since these were all principles I'd worked hard to achieve in my philosophical thinking and writing. It was for me a fairly smooth transition to apply these principles, so useful in orderly thinking, to the physical practice of *asana*, where these very same principles allow the body, over time, to open, unwind, unlock, purify, strengthen, and ultimately achieve some degree of grace and ease through hard work.

Because the mind and body are one, the physical practice of yoga automatically lends itself to a more disciplined way of thinking about how to use the body effectively and respectfully, which includes healthy eating, drinking, and exercise habits, as well as healthy relationships (romantic and otherwise) with others. Yoga can be incredibly revealing in all of these dimensions. It is not 'just exercise,' no, but neither, my husband would tell you, is rock climbing 'just exercise.'[1] And my sister, who competes in mini-triathlons, would certainly deny that those days are 'just exercise' for her. And my brother, who surfed on Maui for five years, would deny that surfing is 'just exercise.' You get the point. There are many, many ways humans have found to move their bodies, breath, and energy in order to feel invigorated, to enjoy the body's full physical capacity, to feel alive. Yoga is one of these ways. I hope that in reading this book you'll come to appreciate the simple insight that yoga is not any one thing. It is something unique and valuable to all of us who practice it and love it enough to write about it in the hope of sharing our

LIZ STILLWAGGON SWAN

own stories about how it has affected our lives. And then maybe you too will give yoga a try, if you haven't already, and discover what it has to offer you.

★★★

In the second part of this introduction, I would like to give you a sense of what insights and stories lie ahead for you to enjoy in this book. The book is divided into four parts: 'Coming into the Space: What is Yoga?,' 'The Asanas: Yoga and the Body,' 'Prana: Yoga's Vital Energy,' and 'Yamas and Niyamas: Ethics and Yoga.' Each part has four or five essays that in one way or another relate to the theme of the section.

The first part, which addresses the big question, 'what is yoga?,' begins with an essay by yoga teacher Jen Munyer, 'How Yoga Won the West,' on the rich and interesting history of yoga. It is a perfect way to begin a book about yoga as it captures the sentiment that yoga has been and is everything you think it is, and more. Munyer traces the rich and deep history of yoga from its origins in around 6500 BCE through its wildly varied permutations, including a stint in the early nineteenth century when it flourished under the guise of traveling circuses in order to escape religious persecution in British-ruled India, to the billion-dollar fitness craze it is today in the West. Munyer's insight into the continually evolving nature of yoga is enriched by her personal experience of coming to yoga in the hopes that it would make her thin and happy, and discovering that it offered not only fitness, health, and happiness, but also so much more.

Next we hear from Kieran McManus who, in 'Will I Find My Guru in India?,' delights us with tales of his recent trip to Nepal and India. McManus explains how, early on in his exotic travels, neither yoga nor India particularly resonated with him, despite his very high expectations. But after finding an amazingly inspiring teacher in Rishikesh – the city made famous in the West when the Beatles spent some time studying transcendental meditation there in the late 1960s – he came to understand and appreciate yoga for the first time in his life: 'I realized that the quality of my yoga session was not about the attainment of challenging poses, but rather the mindfulness of my practice.' McManus explains how with this insight, and several more, he indeed found what he was looking for in India.

In his essay, 'The Seeker,' David Robles addresses the elephant in the yoga studio: Is yoga a religion, a spiritual discipline, or neither? Drawing on his personal experience as co-owner of a yoga studio in multicultural New York state, he explains why more people are discovering the richness of the yogic tradition as they turn away from organized religions while still seeking meaning in their lives. Robles highlights the fact that yoga is very inclusive to people of all religious backgrounds, including the non-religious – a refreshing antidote to the exclusive nature of most traditional religions. Robles' essay also makes the important point that yoga is flexible enough (no pun intended) to remain viable in a scientific world, while ancient religious traditions often have difficulty keeping up with the times.

In their thought-provoking and humorous essay, 'Men, Sports, and Yoga,' Barbara Shaffer and Andrew Purcell ask the provocative question, 'Do real men do yoga?' Nearly eighty percent of all yoga practitioners in the United States (for example) today are women – a curious fact considering that yoga began as a discipline taught and practiced exclusively by men. This essay gives an inside look at three personal stories of men who feel more comfortable pursuing yoga in the privacy of one-on-one sessions with yoga teacher Barbara Purcell than in a group-class setting, which can be intimidating for the uninitiated. Though yoga is commonly touted as being non-competitive, these authors boldly take on the issue and teach us that competition in yoga can come from unexpected places, such as one's ego or one's own bodily limitations.

We end this section with an essay by Steve Jacobson, 'Standing on Your Head, Seeing Things Right Side Up,' who asks the provocative question of whether Westerners, indoctrinated as we are in the rational, scientific tradition of education, are justified in accepting what he calls 'yoga theory.' He explains that yoga theory – which includes everything from *karma* to *chakras* to reincarnation (beliefs from various corners of yoga's long history) – although not completely 'accurate' from a Western perspective, still has some value, in part because some of its wisdom overlaps with that of Western science and medicine. Jacobson concludes that, even if we decide to practice yoga stripped of 'yoga theory,' it is still a very worthwhile practice, perhaps even more so without, as he puts it, all the 'illusion.'

In Part 2 of the book, we turn to the theme of yoga and how it relates to various issues surrounding body awareness and perception. We begin the section with Ken Burak's light-hearted essay, 'Help! My Philosophy Teacher Made Me Touch My Toes!,' which advocates for bringing yoga into the philosophy classroom. As a philosophy teacher, Burak has had great success using yoga to get introductory philosophy students to engage, in a experiential and embodied way, with abstract concepts in philosophy, such as the relations between mind and body, the particular and the universal; the chaotic nature of the human mind; and so on. Burak also explains an insight he has hit upon through this approach to teaching philosophy: the notion that Western philosophy has been one long practice in *pratyahara* (sense withdrawal), which is also, after all, something yogis practice regularly in meditation. Burak proposes that, instead of our maligning Western philosophy for its mistakes and looking to Eastern philosophy for 'solutions,' we should recognize the potential benefits of this long 'retreat' Western philosophy has afforded us, and come to our yoga practice fresh and ready for new insights.

J. Neil Otte's essay, 'Man a Machine, Man a Yogi,' explores the relationship between mind and body as seen in the ancient Eastern texts of the *Yoga Sutras* and the more recent writings of the seventeenth-century philosopher René Descartes and the eighteenth-century physiologist Julien Offray de La Mettrie. Otte suggests that the notion that mind and body are distinct kinds of things, with very different natures, is apparent only in Descartes' analyses, and that both ancient Eastern wisdom and modern materialism see the human mind and body as two functions of the same entity – in other words as united. Otte also delights us with stories of confused proprioception, such as out of body experiences, which he explains can result from yoga practice but nevertheless do not suggest that mind and body are in fact distinct.

We move next to Luna Dolezal's essay, 'Yoga for Women?,' which addresses the deep dissatisfaction that some people, including several essayists in this book, feel concerning how women are portrayed in the yoga world. In the enormously prolific sphere of yoga advertising – in magazines, DVDs, books, and even TV commercials – women who do yoga are portrayed as slim, flexible, and beautiful – often unattainably so. Dolezal takes issue with this particular representation of women especially because, she argues, yoga is supposed to be for everyone. Instead, yoga advertising in the West (particularly the United States) today is stringently exclusive, making potentially the majority of women who might otherwise be drawn to yoga feel inadequate, unwelcome, or not allowed. Dolezal's essay makes an important contribution to the effort of remedying this situation by raising awareness of how bad the situation really is.

In an essay true to its name, 'The Feeling of Beauty,' Nicole Dunas delivers a heartfelt essay about one woman's journey to define what the beautiful is for herself. Disenchanted by how 'beauty' can be so narrowly defined in today's world of anorexic, surgically modified, and airbrushed cover models, Dunas and fellow yoginis decided to pursue a different path with Dunas' creation of The Real Beauty Yoga Project, intended to broaden our conceptualization of what beauty is and how each of us can experience it. Dunas explores some of the historical reasons why even yoga is sometimes guilty of a faddish conceptualization of beauty, and her essay reminds us that beauty is less a way of looking than a way of being.

We conclude this section with Debra Merskin's essay, 'Picturing Yoga,' which provides a systematic analysis of the cover images that have been used for *Yoga Journal* magazine between 2000 and 2008. Merskin explains why the vastly predominant portrayal of the often sexy, almost always white yogini on *Yoga Journal*'s cover is problematic and asks the provocative question of whether a magazine devoted to a historically spiritual discipline ought to be more careful about how it represents itself than the host of other popular magazines that boldly embrace the advertising law that 'sex sells.' Merskin concludes that the tradition in yoga to be inclusive to all types of people – in terms of gender, race, body type, and so on – ought to be reflected by its most widely read pub-lication, *Yoga Journal*.

Part 3 of the book addresses the vital energy, and in some cases healing potential, of yoga. We start with Eric Swan's essay, 'My Guidance Counselor Always Said I'd be a Great Yoga Student,' which addresses an important and topical issue: the role that yoga could play in educational reform in the United States. Swan draws on his ten years of professional experience as a school counselor at the middle- and high-school levels, plus his personal experience of years of regular yoga practice, to reflect on how yoga could enhance students' personal and social development by making them more comfortable with who they are and more confident of their abilities. Swan cites some recent data supporting the idea that yoga in schools could also raise students' academic performance, which is something that public school reform-ers ought to take seriously.

Next we hear from Leigh Duffy, who explains in 'Balance in Yoga and Artistotle' how the concept of balance relates to both the practice of yoga and the philosophy of Aristotle. She shares the story of her terrifying stress-induced collapse, which occurred during the time she was teaching her philosophy students about Aristotle's virtue ethics, wherein a proper balance between extremes is prescribed. The personal crisis helped Duffy to recognize the severe lack of balance in her own life, and this essay describes her journey back to balance through the empowering and steadying practice of yoga. An insight that emerges from this essay is the powerful idea that the balance we try to attain on the mat is only useful when we can bring it into the various other dimensions of our lives.

In 'Healing the Western Mind through Yoga,' Abby Thompson weaves together her expertise in somatic psychology and yoga to make a compelling case for how yoga can be used as an alternative, or supplement, to clinical therapy. She explores the yoga adage, 'how you are on the mat is how you are in life.' For example, she explains how feeling grounded in a balance pose in yoga class can enable one to feel grounded off the mat too, when one is presented with challenges in life. She also enlightens the reader with an interesting connection to neuroscience, explaining that all of our mental and physical habits have a neuronal basis. The good news is that new habits can be established, such as learning to take a deep breath when confronted with stressors and negative emotions.

We conclude this part with an essay in the spirit of the tradition of heart-opening Anusara yoga, wherein, in 'The Path to Happiness Begins with a Journey Inside,' Jim Berti shares with the reader his very personal journey of pain and discontent that led him to the discovery of yoga. Some stories do have a happy ending. Berti tells us that, even in his one year of yoga practice to date, the changes and effects it has had on his personal and professional life have been tremendous. His heartfelt essay reminds all of us who began our practice long ago why we're still finding ourselves on the mat, and will inspire those who have never practiced to consider what yoga could do for them.

The last part of this book opens with an essay by an Iyengar yoga teacher of mine, Jeff Logan, who in his essay 'Get Out of My Way! I'm Late for Yoga!' addresses the philosophical question of whether the yoga teacher has a duty to introduce his or her students to the moral virtues that are so deeply embedded within yogic history and philosophy. Logan delights the reader with both mythological stories from yoga's ancient history and personal stories from his experience as an Iyengar teacher at the studio he co-owns in Huntington, NY. Logan impresses upon the reader just how important it is for students to *live*, rather than simply *know*, yoga philosophy. He gently urges yoga teachers to introduce yoga philosophy to their students by teaching *asanas* (poses) in such a way that they come to embody the very principles of yogic ethical wisdom.

Next, in 'Yoga Off the Mat,' Julinna Oxley explores the transition that every yogi and yogini must make to truly realize his or her yoga practice – that of applying the virtues we practice on the yoga mat, in the yoga studio, to our lives off the mat, outside the yoga studio. She draws on the wisdom of Aristotle's virtue ethics, the essence of which is the insight that being virtuous must come from within rather than from external rules and dogma. Oxley challenges the controversial notion that yogis and yoginis should adopt particular diets or lifestyle habits, arguing that such dictates are not really in the true spirit of yogic, and virtue, ethics, which prescribes more of an internally motivated practice of what it means to be a virtuous person and live a virtuous life.

In Megan Burke's beautifully written and inspiring essay, 'Becoming-Frog,' she shares with the reader her philosophically profound insight that, by practicing the poses of non-human animals as we do in yoga (e.g., frog pose, pigeon pose, and camel pose), we can become more sensitive to the non-human natural environment that contextualizes human life. Burke explains that 'because *asanas* get us out of our habitual way of being in the world as soon as we take on the 'pose' of another creature, we are presented with the possibility of new knowledge.' Her essay draws on the insights of Vandana Shiva's 'Earth democracy' to explain how the very practice of yoga can make one more aware not only of self and others but also of environment and world.

Paul Ulhas MacNeill's essay, 'Yoga and Ethics,' incorporates his twenty years of experience as an ethics professor and a yogi. He credits his yoga practice, rather than his studies and teaching of ethics, with giving him a deep understanding of ethics. MacNeill shares with us some of his deep wisdom of yoga by drawing some interesting comparisons between Eastern and Western perspectives on the origins and role of ethics in our lives. He explains that, with the exception of Aristotle, ethics scholarship in the West has focused largely on intellect and reasoning, whereas in the East the emphasis is on practice, as it is in MacNeill's own life.

The books ends with Heather Salazar's humorously titled essay, 'Why are You Standing on my Yoga Mat?!,' wherein she addresses the not-immediately-apparent connection between one's yoga practice and one's discovery of a 'hidden ethics.' Through a series of insightful and practical exercises, Salazar guides us through an introspective exploration that enables the reader to discover things about herself, such as goals and aspirations, multiple roles in life that may be in conflict, and how to extend the circle of care and concern through some creative partnered yoga exercises. Salazar's essay explains that the actual practice of movement and breath control can help one on the path toward gaining greater self-awareness and becoming more compassionate toward others and toward the world we share with others.

LIZ STILLWAGGON SWAN

It is my hope and intention as editor of this book not only that you will learn something about yoga from this wonderful collection of essays but also that the authors' personal stories about how yoga has touched their lives will delight and inspire you. Happy reading, and *namaste*! (Which, by the way, means that the light within me recognizes and celebrates the light within you!)

NOTE

1 Eric Swan, 'Zen and the art of climbing,' in the *Climbing and Philosophy* book in this series (2010).

ACKNOWLEDGMENTS

I would like to thank, first of all, Eric Swan – loving husband, father of our baby Freeman, fellow yogi (and contributor to this book), and best friend – for his unwavering support in this and all projects I take on in life.

I'd like to acknowledge all of my yoga teachers – past, present, and future – for being sources of inspiration in my yoga practice and in my life. I aspire to have a bit of your yogic wisdom come through in my own teaching.

Heartfelt thanks to John Friend, founder of Anusara yoga, for offering the Foreword to the book, and to all the contributors for their beautiful and insightful essays about yoga, from which I have learned so much. I look forward to practicing yoga with you someday, somewhere. *Namaste*!

Thank you to Fritz Allhoff for his enthusiasm about this book from the very beginning, and a special thanks to the Wiley-Blackwell team: to Jeff Dean for suggesting the subtitle, and to Tiffany Mok and Hazel Harris for their guidance throughout the planning and execution of the book.

And, last but certainly not least, to the wonderful people at the Center for the Humanities at Oregon State University, where, during the 2010–2011 academic year, I had a cozy office, lots of time, and an unlimited supply of coffee to work on this and other writing projects. Long live the Horning Endowment, and go Beavers.

Liz Stillwaggon Swan

PART I

COMING INTO THE SPACE:
WHAT IS YOGA?

CHAPTER I

HOW YOGA WON THE WEST

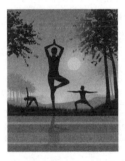

In the Beginning...

'Will yoga make me thin and happy?' Thus, my path of yoga began. I didn't find yoga because I was interested in union with some divine ultimate reality. I wasn't a philosophy or religious studies student searching for answers to the existential nature of my being. I didn't stumble onto the path of yoga because I happened to be born into a family who practiced it. I didn't even know I was looking for yoga. I was a depressed and overweight twenty-one-year-old searching for a way to get thin, because I believed that was the key to my happiness. At the time I worked in a flower shop and a woman there befriended me. She watched me struggle with myself and after a few weeks asked whether I had ever tried yoga. I answered no and asked her my most important question: would it make me thin and happy? Now, a decade later, every time I step on my mat, I offer gratitude to my first teacher, Ute, whose response to that question was: You never know what will unfold when you step on the mat.

What brought you to your mat for the first time? And, if you have yet to step on a mat, what kinds of curiosities lead you to pick up this book?

Yoga – Philosophy for Everyone: Bending Mind and Body, First Edition.
Edited by Liz Stillwaggon Swan.
© 2012 John Wiley & Sons, Inc. Published 2012 by John Wiley & Sons, Inc.

Today, it seems like yoga is the solution to everything. We hear doctors telling us it's good for our health; psychologists say it's good for our emotional well-being; yoga teachers talk about union with something bigger than the human experience; gurus talk about alternative states of consciousness; and perhaps your friends have shared with you how yoga has changed their lives. Can a practice really do all of that? With all these different experiences of it, and prescriptions of why to use it, what is yoga anyway?

Throughout the history of humankind, we have attempted, in myriad ways, to answer three questions: Who am I? Where did I come from? How should I live my life? When I was searching for the key to my happiness, unconsciously I was in the throes of trying to answer these questions. Up until that point in my life, I had searched for the answers to those questions everywhere, except within myself. I was so used to looking to my parents for answers, or to academia, to the church, or to what my peers were doing, that I never stopped to think that, if I could learn to listen to that faint whisper inside myself, I would have my own answers to those questions.

Stepping on the Mat

When I stood on my mat for the first time, I experienced anger, frustration, sadness, curiosity, overwhelming peace, silence, and an inner critic with an incredibly loud voice. I know: a lot was happening! Despite the crowd of voices and experiences, what really happened on the mat was that for the first time I *witnessed* the entirety of what was happening inside of me. And because I could witness it, another part of me awoke – an aspect of myself that had incredible compassion, tolerance, and patience for the part of me that was hurting.

As I reached for my toes (intent on going further into the stretch than anyone else in the room) and my hamstrings sung out in defiance, for a brief moment I was able to make a connection between how hard I was pushing myself to 'look the best' in the pose and how hard I was pushing myself in life to live up to some idealized version of me. That awareness only lasted a moment, but it was enough to bring me back to my mat, again and again. I was hooked; I wanted to know why bending forward to touch my toes brought up such a large inner experience. And what was it about being aware of my body in this way that allowed me to *witness*

JENNIFER MUNYER

my thoughts and feelings, instead of unconsciously and habitually reacting to them? What was it about the practice that brought forth that witnessing consciousness? Ute was right: There is no telling what will unfold when I am being present with myself, and being on the mat teaches me that.

It is this mystery of myself that has kept me going for the past decade. After that first class, I knew yoga was about much more than twisting my body into a pretzel. I had a sense it was about something much bigger even than losing weight. There was a resonance with something bigger than me, a sensation that felt oddly familiar. It was the sensation I once had of the Holy Spirit. It was the same sensation I felt after a long, exhausting climb to the top of a mountain. It was the same depth of silence I felt after a fresh snowfall. That sensation was there in the last gaze my grandma ever gave me. It has been called many names throughout the course of human history, and, whatever it is, I recognized that something about presence and reaching for my toes allowed me to experience it, within myself, again.

The Exploration of Yoga

As yoga becomes more and more mainstream in the West, there are more and more attempts to define and explain what this ancient practice is. To some people it is a hippie movement, to others a cult religion, and to still others a new fad in the exercise industry. There are numerous commentaries on the practice, a multitude of scholastic research papers and books, several scientific studies on its physical effects, and myriad individual stories about its personal effects. More often than not, the more visible something becomes, the more questions there are about it. Many of my new students ask questions like: 'I'm not really flexible, can I still do yoga?' 'Will practicing yoga make my stress go away?' and 'Why can't I breathe deeply?'

Western culture tends to like answers, looking for physical proof and experiencing trepidation about trusting the unknown. Further, Westerners tend to thrive on experience, sensations, and a depth of curiosity that drives us toward creative endeavors. It makes sense that the majority of Westerners want to know a bit about what they are going to do before they do it. And learning a bit about yoga philosophy before, or while, engaging with a practice is supportive of a fuller embodiment of the practice. The benefits of yoga are greatly enhanced when there is an understanding of the intention (and philosophy) behind it. I hope this essay will offer you some explanations of the ever-evolving nature of yoga, evoke further curiosity about what it is, and shed light on how this current form of yoga is both the same and different from its traditional roots.

It's All a Matter of Perspective

Over thousands of years, as the practice of yoga has moved from culture to culture, the expression and perception of yoga have changed several times. There are undeniable core truths to the philosophy and practice of yoga, and as it moves between cultures and continents the practice is flexible enough to use the current language and cultural consciousness to adapt its image. Just as you might dress up for a wedding or down for pizza night while who you are remains intact, yoga may be dressed differently in each culture, or in each tradition, while its core remains the same. Modern definitions and attempts to explain the path of yoga are filtered through cultural and individual experience.

While this essay might offer you a general overview of how yoga became what it is today, keep in mind that the explanations I offer come through the filter of my own experience. While you might read all about yoga from others' perspectives, stepping onto your mat will reveal your own mystery and give you a deeper meaning of yoga than I, or any other author, might be able to provide for you. As the great teacher K. Pattabhi Jois used to say, 'Practice, practice, practice. Ninety-nine percent practice. One percent theory.' My hope is that, as a result of reading this essay, a spark of curiosity will be lit and you will take it upon yourself to seek out your own experience of yoga.

The filter of experience through which you will be reading comes from a white, middle-class, fourth-generation-American female, who has spent only a decade of her life in self-study (*svadhyaya*), practice (*tapas*), and letting go to something bigger than her (*ishvara pranidhanani*). Almost all of the teachers I have had the privilege of learning from learned from someone who learned from someone who trained with a teacher in India. My path of yoga is unique to me, and has provided me with opportunities to experience some of the depth of what yoga is ultimately translated as: union.

JENNIFER MUNYER

The Birth of Yoga

In its most literal translation, yoga means 'to yoke' or 'to unite.' A broad, encompassing definition refers to the joining together of one's physical experience with universal energy. To gather a sense of what this means, let's start at the beginning and explore the historical roots of yoga. Perhaps reading the story of the evolution of this practice will provide some insight into how our innate human urge to understand and unite with the unknown took shape in what became called the practice of yoga. Perhaps this way of telling the story will enable you to see the ever-evolving nature of yoga, and how its essence has stayed the same while its form has changed to meet the demands of each evolving time period.

The first sign of anything that resembled what we now think of as yoga was an emblem on a business-card-like impression called the Pashupati seal. Imagine the body of a man, sitting in *padmasana* (lotus position: legs crossed with ankles by hip creases), wearing a striped tunic, a mask, and a huge headdress in the shape of two large horns. The Pashupati seal was created in the Indus Valley in around 6500 BCE, a period known as the Pre-Vedic Age. The Pre-Vedic Age encompassed the time period before the written word (which meant that the only way to pass anything on was through symbols and oral recitation), before traditionally recognized religions such as Hinduism, and at a time in human history when we were connected (or united) with nature in a way that is now mostly foreign to us.

In part because there was not yet any written language, there were many great and layered meanings behind symbols such as the Pashupati seal. In lieu of written narratives, these symbols held rich stories within their images. Perhaps this was the beginning of the long history of using symbolism to describe experiences that seem to be indescribable. Using symbols allowed each person to pass on both the well-defined rituals of a yoga practice and the personal (story-like) experiences embedded within the teachings. One of the stories of this seal had to do with the image of Shiva, an aspect of divine consciousness, who sat in the woods to expound upon a path that would lead individuals to divine realization. This particular symbol of Shiva spoke of being in union with both his higher and lower natures and is the platform for many of the yogic rituals of meditation that seek to bring unity between the human and divine aspects of oneself.

What does 'Divine' Mean to You?

It feels prudent to take a moment to pause in this history to define what I mean when I say 'divine.' When I use the word 'divine,' I am speaking about a great mystery – about an ineffable experience humans are incapable of describing with words. Because divine experience is beyond description, the divine has been embodied into forms so that it is easier to speak about and relate to. As humans, we use form, whether that is words, symbols, or movements, to communicate with one another. Experiences that go beyond words necessitate form. The form, as a symbol of the ineffable experience, may then be used to speak about the ineffable experience. When I mention the divine throughout this essay I am referring to whatever symbol or form you might use to describe your experience of something that feels indescribable to you.

In human history, we have tried several different ways to speak about these kinds of experience. This is evidenced by the numerous religions and philosophies that all attempt to give form and name to the eternal essence that is the common thread through them all. This is what has happened with yoga. Its essence remains unchanged, while its form has evolved throughout history. Yoga's essence adapts to fit the familiar symbols in each culture and time period.

A New Era Begins...

After the Pre-Vedic Age, the written word was developed. From this time period, known as the Vedic Age, several important evolutionary steps in yoga occurred. At this time, those adept at practicing and guiding others along the path of yoga were not the priests but the rishis and sages. They were people who lived in union (in yoga) in nature. They took a natural way of life and modeled a discipline after it that came to be known as yoga. Their teachings led to the first glimpses of how internal inquiry could guide an individual on the path of living in union with the divine. Their wisdom was written and became known as the Vedas.

The study of the Vedas is non-dual, meaning that the Vedas explain the inherent nature of the divine within physical experience. There is no separation (no dualistic relationship) between this reality and the divine.

There are four main texts that make up the Vedas – the *Rigveda*, *Yajurveda*, *Samaveda*, and *Atharyaveda*. The Vedas were regarded as a form of sacred knowledge – thus rendering the actual Sanskrit words as sacred themselves. These texts spelled out the proper performance of sacrifices and rituals while also recording incantations meant to bring about union with the divine.

For thousands of years, humans had been living in union with nature, learning from it and communing with it. Humans who were sensitive to the ways of the Earth (e.g., the seasons, cycles, and patterns) and those who were able to spend time contemplating their existence within nature had cultivated great experiential wisdom from yoga. These abilities and practices had been passed down the generations through spoken word and symbols alone. Then, the advent of the written word made available the ability to write down these ancient secrets and practices. Thus the recorded history of yoga began.

The Vedic Age was also the beginning of what we now know in the yoga world as *mantra*. *Mantra* is the painstaking memorization and recitation of the exact tone and enunciation of the Vedic scriptures, and is used by a path of yoga we have come to know as Japa yoga. In this form the divine makes itself known through the devotion of precise recitation. Japa yoga is integral to the devotional form of yoga known as Bhakti yoga. Cultivated by reciting the Vedas, performing and attending ritual sacrifices, and through the devotional practice of Bhakti yoga, these now-familiar ideas of what yoga is associated with emerged in the Vedic time period: concentration, watchfulness, austerity, watching the breath (meditation), and devotion. Spiritual life flourished in the Vedic Age.

What Goes Up Must Come Down

The essence of evolution is being able to adapt to environmental change. As change is inherent in life, what adapts well will survive. Have you ever noticed that, after a while, when it feels like your life is flourishing, a challenge comes along, oftentimes wiping out the feelings of prosperity? This is also a pattern in the larger picture of life: there is a pattern of golden ages, followed by dark ages, followed by rebuilding in middle ages, only to allow for more golden ages, and so on. Throughout these natural cycles of life and death, birth and rebirth, that which remains is that which is best able to adapt to the changes, and therefore evolves and thrives.

Marking the end of the prosperous Vedic Age around 500 BCE, a war began that would later become known through the great Indian epic, the *Mahabarata*. This war, between two ruling families, plunged India into its Dark Ages. Consider what happens for you when life becomes dark, uncertain, or terrifying. I know that, when I fall into that kind of experience in my life, my tendency is to cling to what feels solid and secure. The ways in which the people responded to The Great War were not so different. During the centuries that followed, known as the Brahmanical Age, priests (or brahmans) became the elite class. They became the primary advisers to the ruling class and used their rhetoric on religious teachings to encourage a very strict ritualistic approach towards governing. The performance of rituals and sacrifice was an exact science and taken to be literal. Only people of the brahman class could perform rituals or seek out the sacred texts. The brahmans systematized the Vedas. The rishis and sages no longer had large influence, but instead became part of the fringes of society – *sannyasins* (hermits) living in the forest.

The path taken by this fringe group diverged. One group continued to live on the outskirts but stayed connected with the Vedic teachings of the time. They wrote a sacred text known as the *Aranyakas* (forest teachings) and paved the way for the Upanishads. They still engaged in rituals, but the focus of these rituals was on the internal nature of sacrifice.

The other half continued to explore the ancient rites in a non-orthodox way. They formed a band of nomads that became known as the Vrratya Brothers and traveled around, exploring sex, magic, breath, and subtle energy. In contrast to the brahman class, which gave highest recognition to the masculine energy of the divine, the Vrratya Brothers gave more credence and reverence to the feminine forms of energy. This fringe of society helped to seed the roots of a well-developed lineage of yoga today, known as tantric yoga.

While it was beginning to take on several different forms, yoga's essence – union with the great mystery of life – still lived on in these different expressions. The essence of yoga (concentration, mindfulness, present moment attention, and union with the divine) lived on through all these different expressions. It would be easy to say that, because the teachings looked different, it was no longer yoga. But that would be like saying that, because you look different at age eighty from how you looked at birth, you are no longer you.

A Shift in Perspective

The Post-Vedic Age was populated with a diverse group of people. With such diversity, and the myriad ways to explore the ancient traditions, an ideological revolution occurred. While the brahmans were still the elite class, their perception of yoga evolved. This path was now being explored with more esoteric wisdom and transcendental knowledge. As opposed to external sacrifices, inner worship and meditative practices abounded. This revolution of thought, based on previous centuries of differing experiences, had an atmosphere that encouraged exploration of the unknown. The Upanishads, more sacred texts of yogic philosophy, were the product of this revolution.

As wisdom is gained through experience, concepts become clarified and unfold in deeper meaning. While the Upanishads were radically different from the Vedas, they were not a departure from them, but rather an evolution. The Upanishads made explicit what the Vedas had hinted at. Whereas the Vedas hinted at the mystery of form, the Upanishads wrote that behind the reality of multiple forms exists an unchanging single being. The Upanishads allowed for difference in form with the recognition of that form as one expression of a single, united, divine consciousness. The Upanishads also held that access to the divine comes purely from inside; while helpful, no external means of accessing the divine are necessary.

Four concepts from the Post-Vedic Age connected the past with what would become the future of yoga. Within these four concepts ring the tones of early Pre-Vedic worship and the forms of Buddhism and Jainism (two religions that formed out of this time period's influence) that were yet to come. The four concepts are:

- Innermost nature is a total mirror of outermost nature and is called *atman* (or, in the West, self).
- Realization of self and ultimate reality frees us from suffering.
- Thoughts and actions determine what is to come (destiny) and *karma* is becoming what you identify with.
- Unless one is liberated and achieves ultimate reality, one will be reborn (laying out, for the first time, a clarification of reincarnation).

The Pre-Classical Age took these four concepts and extrapolated upon them in a few different ways. Six schools of philosophy emerged; both

Buddhism and Jainism were born; and the great Indian epics, the *Ramayana* and the *Mahabarata*, were written. These great epics were a classical example of a return to using story and symbol to bring forth a message. Their contents offer examples of 'right action' by demonstrating moral disciplines and wisdom over action through their characters' adventures.

The Father of Modern Yoga

The Classical Age (100 BCE to 500 CE) is the next stop in this story. This was when what the West knows as yoga and all that came before began to merge. Somewhere in this time period, a sage called Patañjali wrote the first book outlining, in simple terms, practical ways for the common person to access the royal path of yoga, Raja yoga, in the *Yoga Sutras* of Patañjali.

There are many outstanding commentaries on the *Yoga Sutras*, so I will refrain from going into very much depth about them here. In short, the *Yoga Sutras* of Patañjali outline methods to still the mind. In book two of the *Sutras*, Patañjali writes about the eight limbs of Raja yoga. He expresses that, since the body and mind are inseparable, both must learn how to become still in order to sense the subtle expressions, the quiet whispers, of the divine. *Asana* (postures) and *pranayama* (breath control) are but two of the eight limbs that aid an individual in bringing stillness to his or her being. This is the first mention in the history of yoga of the reason for postural practice.

The Cycle Repeats Itself

What does all this history have to do with how yoga is shaping a sphere of influence in the West? While it may not look the same every time, history does repeat itself. Once again, yoga was flourishing. Its influence in the East grew for many centuries. The aforementioned six schools of Indian philosophy (one of which was yoga) were born out of this history. The fringe group that seeded the roots for tantra grew ever more discerning with their study of subtle energy and the divine feminine energy. Further expositions on yoga (which had more of an emphasis on postural practice), such as the *Hatha Yoga Pradipika*, were written to clarify aspects of Patañjali's *Yoga Sutras*. By the Post-Classical Age (1300–1700), India had risen out of the Dark and Middle Ages and found herself flourishing again, in a way reminiscent of the Vedic Age. But then, with the invasion and colonization of India by the British in the early nineteenth century, yoga was once again asked to survive the challenge of change, and evolve.

In the early years of British rule, yoga and the forms it took were greatly discouraged and looked down upon. In response, yoga went underground. This time its practitioners did not only go to the forests; they also found a way to keep the practice alive under the guise of entertainment. An inspired yoga practitioner named T. S. Krishnamacharya formed traveling 'circuses' – demonstrations of the physical aspect of yoga. While these were often seen as entertainment by the ruling classes, the ancient line of yogic philosophy and practice was being passed on to the students of these traveling exhibitions. Once again, yoga found a way to adapt, evolve, and continue its influence.

Over time these displays of great physical ability were brought to Europe, where traditional *asanas* were mixed with the dynamic flowing forms of European calisthenics, which still have great influence on how Westerners view yoga practice today. In 1893, Swami Vivekananda, an intensely brilliant young man with a deep desire to transmit the message of unity through multiplicity, traveled to Chicago to address the Parliament of Religions. His teachings were some of the very first yogic teachings to and gain respect from people in the United States. Unlike how yoga is currently viewed in the West, Vivekananda's teachings had nothing to do with twisting bodies into pretzels. Instead, his message carried the essence of yogic teachings about union through encouraging peace, unity, and compassion. As Westerners grew interested in yoga, some began traveling to India to study with teachers such as Krishnamacharya, his son T. K. V. Desikachar, son-in-law B. K. S. Iyengar, and esteemed student K. Pattabhi Jois.

How Yoga Won the West

While yoga was being practiced among the wealthy as early as the late 1800s in the United States, Krishnamacharya's first female student, Indra Devi, is credited with making yoga popular in the United States. Similarly to how Krishnamacharya used yoga's physical component to attract new students, Devi emphasized yoga's benefit to personal health. This has contributed to the evolution of yoga as we know it in the West. There are more branches on the family tree of yoga than ever before. While yoga may take on many forms, they are all born from the same tree.

My path to yoga began with the question, 'Will it make me thin and happy?,' and I am forever grateful for the introduction of yoga for physical benefit in the West. But, as you have just read, there is quite a bit more to yoga than being able to twist your body into a pretzel. One philosophical concept in the *Yoga Sutras* is that there is a differentiation between layers of consciousness. This can be likened to the following analogy: Consider the various forms water may take – liquid, solid and gas. The solid state is the easiest to discern, to become aware of, and, as your ability to perceive with your senses deepens, so does your sensitivity in discerning the multitude of ranges between solids, liquids, and gases.

Perhaps, then, it makes sense that Western culture would need to be introduced to yoga in its densest form – that is, under the guise of its being a physical practice. No matter how yoga is known, no matter what form it takes in Western culture, yoga is ever-evolving. It will adapt and find expression in a way that makes sense to the society and culture of each era. This does not take away from the unchanging essence of yoga. Behind the multiplicity of forms lies a single, unchanging truth. There is unity within different forms. This is the ever-evolving nature of yoga.

JENNIFER MUNYER

CHAPTER 2

WILL I FIND MY GURU IN INDIA?

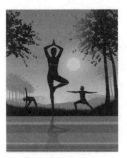

My decision to quit my job and travel the world came at a junction in my life. I was single, didn't have kids or a mortgage, and was bored silly at my job. I was at rope's end and felt that my creative soul had fallen asleep. My fire was dimmed low, and I found myself in a dull place in life most of Monday through Friday. I was seeking something but I couldn't put my finger on what. I wanted to feel alive, to feel like my life had significance and that moments were inspired by divine meaning. The words of the Persian poet Hafiz haunted me: 'I am the flute through which the Christ's breath flows.' I wanted to feel that way.

One night a vision spontaneously exploded in my mind. I decided that I would quit my job and begin truly following my heart. For many years I had been dreaming of a journey around Asia to explore music, cultures, and peoples. Through most of those years I feared it would never happen. But now the time seemed right and there was nothing to hold me back. The yearning in my heart was so strong that I knew that I had to do it. For the first time in a long while, I was ecstatic to be alive. Everything felt right.

Yoga – Philosophy for Everyone: Bending Mind and Body, First Edition.
Edited by Liz Stillwaggon Swan.
© 2012 John Wiley & Sons, Inc. Published 2012 by John Wiley & Sons, Inc.

Over the next few weeks I sold my car and most of my possessions. What remained I put in storage. I felt perfectly liberated, free to follow my heart. The East was calling me. Something was waiting for me there. I spent many nights in bed wide-eyed and restless, confident that a breakthrough was waiting for me. Maybe it was love, maybe I would discover my calling in life, maybe I would find my guru.

The Winding Road to India

The journey was loosely scripted and nothing was cast in stone. I didn't even know which countries I would visit, nor how long my trip would last. I bought a one-way ticket to Nepal with a general plan of eventually making it to Thailand. The overarching goal of the journey was to be fully present at all times. I wanted to be in that place where my path was constantly being guided by divine suggestion.

My lofty dreams about the East were shaken soon after the plane touched down in Nepal. Kathmandu is Nepal's biggest city and, while it is a place of fascinating culture and profound beauty, it is also a crowded, crazy city of pollution and honking cars. I was hoping to find peace and happiness, but I was in the heart of chaos. I quickly realized that finding happiness and peace couldn't be dependent on my environment. I needed to find peace within my self.

After a few months of constant movement, I was tired and found myself considering my travels from a different perspective. I had been studying the Lonely Planet guidebook intensely and had visited many temples, trekked through the Himalayas, explored many cities, and rented motorcycles on which to buzz around visiting tourist attractions. I had met many great people and had countless wonderful experiences. But something was still missing. Reflecting on my days back in the office, I found myself still trying to understand the critical question, 'What am I looking for?'

For me, part of the intrigue of traveling is experiencing what I can't find at home. One of the things that had led me to come East in the first place was my desire to find spiritual guidance. Sure, there are churches and wise people everywhere, but as I traveled, over and over, I heard people describing their experiences in India. Their descriptions filled my mind with great visions. They spoke of the myriad ashrams and monasteries where enlightened teachers instructed those who came to learn.

They spoke of the sadhus, mystics, yogis, and wandering monks that have called India home for thousands of years. Through all of their stories I was hearing clear confirmation that India should be my destination. While I really hadn't been planning on visiting India, and despite my secret fears of such a chaotic country, all of these surreal descriptions of India's spiritual heart convinced me that, on this great journey, I needed to go there. I thought I would only stay a month or two. Given India's reputation for profound over-population and general pandemonium I suspected I wouldn't want to stay much longer. But I was wrong.

Crossing the border from Nepal into India, I witnessed just how tumultuous India is. It was an exciting kind of tumult, though. The first place I visited was Varanasi, a bustling city in northern India along the shores of the holy Ganga river. Its narrow stone corridors were busy with pilgrims, cows, dogs, and tourists. There were many temples and shrines in the area and all along the river religious rituals were taking place. Morning, noon, and night, several towers of black smoke rose up from funeral pyres where the deceased were being cremated. Despite the turbulent environment, I was struck by the intensity of the Indian devotional fervor. The spiritual presence was tangible.

In the weeks that followed, India's lure wrapped its arms around me and held me tightly. The days were long and amazing, filled with countless strange and spontaneous adventures, experiences, and peoples. The landscape was varied and beautiful, the food was incredible, and every day I had great experiences with inspirational people in chance situations.

Many Masters, Many Roads

Traveling in India is tourism unlike that found anywhere else in the world. There seems to be a certain sort of folk traveling there. Many come with spiritual inclinations and India offers everything they are seeking. The traveler circuit is abuzz with myriad schools of diverse spiritual traditions, including offerings in yoga, meditation, reiki, tai chi, Buddhism, Hinduism, and ayurveda. In the course of my travels, I encountered many travelers asking interesting questions, seeking a better understanding of themselves and God, and wondering how their lives were relevant in the grand cosmic picture. I was surprised to find that most travelers were like me, coming to India with hopes of studying with enlightened masters. It excited me greatly to think that there still exists a place on Earth where great teachers can be found carrying on the unbroken lineage of ancient wisdom, preserved in an oral tradition, from teacher to student.

Of all the spiritual hotspots along the traveler's circuit, Rishikesh stood out as a common favorite. I naïvely suspected Rishikesh had become popular because the Beatles spent time there in 1967 while studying Transcendental Meditation. But, as I did more research, I learned that Rishikesh means 'land of the sages' and has been for many centuries a holy place where spiritual aspirants have come for prayer, meditation, and yoga at its many mountain shrines and ashrams. After five months of traveling around Nepal and India, Rishikesh suddenly seemed like the perfect answer to my soul's prayer. I wanted to be still and immerse myself in meditation and spiritual inquiry.

After a long, harrowing bus ride north from Delhi, I arrived in Rishikesh. My first impressions were of pretty typical Indian city. Cows and dogs were milling about chaotic streets crowded with honking cars, pedestrians, and rickshaws. But then I crossed over a cable footbridge into the spiritual heart of Rishikesh. Surrounded by Himalayan mountains, I stood beside the icy green Ganga river surveying the surreal landscape. Magical Rishikesh and all of her temples and shrines were unfolding before me. As I walked along, I loved it immediately. There was no doubt in my mind that I'd be there a while.

Everywhere I went I saw young, fit travelers walking around with yoga mats slung over their shoulders. I soon learned that Rishikesh is the 'world capital of yoga' and has many yoga schools offering various flavors of instruction. This intrigued me immensely since I had been wanting to experience traditional yoga in its purest form.

I asked around town and learned of classes with noteworthy teachers. There were many, and so I began sampling them. But in each class, I found myself attempting to keep up with the others while lacking an understanding of why I was doing these strange things with my body. I felt hopeless, like yoga would never be for me. I looked around the room and saw everyone holding challenging postures effortlessly. Then there was newbie me, clueless, probably making every mistake in the book. I felt like an idiot and was frustrated by my lack of understanding. I just didn't get yoga. However, as Rishikesh was such a carnival of spiritual wonderment, even if the yoga thing didn't work out, I was happy to find other ways to spend my days in this enchanted village.

While there, I stayed at the Sri Ved Niketan Ashram. This ashram, like many around India, served dual purposes. It was a guesthouse as well as a place for spiritual inquiry. I had always had an interest in Hinduism, and this particular ashram offered daily mediation sessions as well as lectures on Vedic philosophy. I was greatly intrigued and began attending the ashram's offerings as soon as I got there.

Classes were led by the ashram's spiritual director, a curious man named Swami Dharmananda. He could be found every morning in the meditation cave sitting in darkness, meditating. Two dozen framed portraits of yogis and saints ranging from Jesus to Shiva adorned the altar at the front of the room. Between ten and twenty Western and Indian meditators were usually gathered around Swami Dharmananda, sitting in near darkness with just a dim candle burning. Rising well before sunrise in the still of the night, we would gather every morning to learn various techniques for stilling and sharpening the mind.

Swami Dharmananda's lectures were always incredibly interesting, as he conveyed the intricacies of Hinduism with precision and decisiveness. He explained that the *Bhagavad Gita* was the fruit of many wise people searching for truth. It had an organic authorship in that it was the result of knowledge acquired by many searchers through the centuries. Swami Dharmananda spoke in depth about yoga, one of the practices that evolved under this comprehensive system. He explained that one's diet and actions affect the spiritual body. I was very intrigued by this concept – it made so much sense to me. Swami Dharmananda also lectured about yoga's importance in traditional Hinduism, as it provides a framework of meditation, practices, and ethics necessary for self-realization. His lectures intensified my desire to connect with yoga. But still I hadn't found the right teacher.

And then divine intervention happened.

Spiritual Boot Camp

One day I walked into a riverside café and bumped into a friend I'd met a few months earlier in Nepal. I took a seat and we began discussing our time in Rishikesh so far. I mentioned my inability to find the right yoga class. Like a cosmic messenger, he instantly launched into a description of the Agama Yoga School, where he had just completed a program.

With great enthusiasm he explained how the school received students as a complete beginner and gave them a foundational understanding of yogic theory, *chakras*, and the body's energy channels. The course was a four-week intensive program that combined lectures with *asana* (postures) practice, providing students with a solid grasp of the components that make the yogi's life a powerful spiritual discipline.

Listening to my friend describe this yoga program, I knew this was the doorway into the yoga experience I had been looking for. And, when he mentioned the next course would be starting the following morning, there was no doubt in my mind that I was supposed to be there.

The next day I got up early and, after morning meditation with Swami Dharmananda, headed off to my first day of yoga class. On my clunky Indian bicycle, I rode down the stone path beside the Ganga river, weaving in and out of cows and street dogs and excrement and sadhus scattered along the roads. I found the school at the back of a temple. The classroom was a concrete room with nothing more than two dozen yoga mats and pictures of yogis and saints on the walls.

I found a mat at the front of the room and closed my eyes for a moment of gratitude and prayed for an open mind. I really wanted to understand how yoga could improve my physical and spiritual life. At the front of the room there was a beautiful Indian man dressed in white, deep in meditation. At half past eight on the dot, he opened his eyes, stood up, and began teaching.

He was instantly captivating. He was an intense and incredibly intriguing human being, and I just wanted to listen to him. His name was Kushru, and, as he spoke, every word found a home in my heart. In my whole life I had never had a teacher that had captured my attention more powerfully. His piercing focus never wavered, and he held every single student in the palm of his hand as we listened attentively and processed every word he spoke.

With conviction and eloquence, Kushru instructed us about the wisdom accumulated over hundreds of years by countless spiritual aspirants. His lectures merged Indian Vedanta with Western scientific medical findings, philosophy, poetry, and music, creating a patchwork of wisdom gathered from various disciplines throughout the centuries. Even more impressive than his words was his confidence and self-understanding. Clearly, Kushru benefited from the method he was teaching. He was a teacher in the truest sense of the word. He inspired students through his example.

The first week of class was mostly theoretical, with only a few short sessions of *asana* practice. Kushru explained how yoga puts the mind and body in resonance with the universe. Devoid of New-Age-speak and clichés, which always bore me, Kushru's teachings spanned a wide range of topics, including morality, *karma*, hygiene, diet, willpower, and meditation.

What began as a simple desire to learn *asanas* evolved into a much larger practice of purifying and managing my mind so that my physical body could become a sacred vehicle. Kushru's lectures were riveting and every day I left class feeling like I'd been granted a golden key to understanding.

I was fascinated by the yogic concept of purifying the body and mind through yoga and meditation so as to acquire a healthy balance with the universe. The result of such a practice, Kushru explained, could be seen in the lives of India's many great yogis. He told us incredible anecdotes of yogis whose lives were spent in complete devotion to God. He spoke of yogis who were known to have performed supernatural feats, such as levitating, or appearing in multiple places simultaneously, or having the uncanny ability to see the future and knowing things of which they had no experience. He spoke of Ramakrishna, who had spent six months in quasi-lifeless meditation before being conditioned back to life. After all these stories, Kushru offered the summary that, when we become masters of our minds, we exist on a spiritual level where we can actually transcend physical laws.

In the West, many of us are raised looking to Jesus as the one, singular, godly figure of awe who walked on water, defied death, and made miracles happen simply by willing them. These stories made a believer out of me a long time ago, but I never realized that in India these feats are not that extraordinary. Over the course of thousands of years, India has produced many yogis known to have attained enlightenment and self-mastery, with the ability to achieve feats that we in the West call miracles.

The course was designed to encourage us to always be mindful of the spiritual gains of each *asana*. We learned one new *asana* every day. Our instructors demonstrated the physical posture and then imparted a thorough understanding of how each *asana* affected the *chakras* and energy channels. When it came time to practice, we held each *asana* for several minutes, allowing us to sink into a deep state of concentration. The *asanas*, for the first time in my life, began to resonate with me. I finally felt like I got it – I realized that the quality of my yoga session was not about the attainment of challenging poses, but rather the mindfulness of my practice.

Breaking Through

During the month-long yoga course, the days were long and intense. Between Kushru's mind-bending lectures and the demanding *asana* sessions, I was being challenged to reach further into my heart. Sometimes the physical discomfort seemed intolerable, but I was being challenged to recognize sensations as neutral that our minds naturally characterize as positive or negative. This was hardcore soul-work for me, but I liked it. And, though there were many days when I'd return to my ashram broken and exhausted, I was happy. My life was changing, as the course spoke directly to my heart.

With each new day, I began to see how yoga, while not necessarily a religion, is a physical discipline that connects us with our sacred core. It applies scientific truths upon the body as the yogi purifies and strengthens the body and mind. Reflecting on Kushru's teaching on *karma*, I was inspired by the notion that every single thing we do, say, and think either brings us closer to, or further away from, our ultimate goal of attaining our sacred potential.

Zing! That was it. That was the missing piece. I needed to better understand the sacred life force within all of us. My yoga practice had effectively conveyed the notion that mindfulness and intention define our experience in life. Suddenly this concept seemed obvious to me and I realized I had found what I was looking for. There would always be hardship, suffering, and misfortune in my live, but the yogi transcends negative experience by remaining in the sacred place where all experience is an opportunity for spiritual growth.

A New Day

By the final week of the course, I felt like a new person. I felt like a yogi! I was practicing *asanas* with mindfulness and attention to the spiritual experience. I was training to channel and promote positive energy flow throughout the body. I had accepted the fact that living a truly moral life is a prerequisite to spiritual maturity, and that the concept of *karma* is unavoidable. The importance of generosity had been underscored. My perception had been expanded from a miniature view of the self as an individual in a disconnected world to one of the self's potential as a complete perfect system, a smaller version of the universe.

I began to understand how all religions lead to the same place. Every tradition's teachings explain a method through which a practitioner becomes pure and lives in harmony with self and others. Yogic philosophy, like all the great religions, presents an order of the world where the individual is part of the cosmic whole. But, unlike most religious teachings, the yogi's methods are devoid of dogma and jargon. Yoga is simply the science of self-understanding and mastery, which allows one to be happy and live meaningfully.

After my rewarding stay in Rishikesh, I knew in my heart that my journey had come to an end. I felt like the flute Hafiz spoke of, through which the Christ's breath flows. I knew I had a lot of work ahead of me as I continued to fine-tune the *asanas* and internalize the teachings I had learned, but I knew that, whether I was in India or the United States, I was exactly where I needed to be. And that place was good.

CHAPTER 3

THE SEEKER

How Yoga is Meeting Changing Western Spiritual Needs

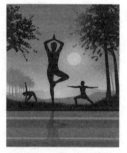

The religious landscape of the United States, along with that of the rest of the Western world, is changing. The change is subtle, pervasive, and, to some, worrisome. More and more people are rejecting the religion of their parents, while some find meaning in other traditions, grafting them onto their native doctrines. Others refuse to identify with any traditional religion and instead create a personalized hodge-podge of beliefs from any number of sources, defining themselves as 'spiritual' rather than religious. It is as if the walls separating religions are crumbling. I see it every day in my yoga classes. There is the Christian who believes in reincarnation, the Jewish woman who believes in *karma*, and the atheist who feels a profound sense of peace in meditation, all sitting together on their mats chanting 'om.'

Some worry that this trend represents a movement away from traditional religious values, and others celebrate what they perceive as the decline of religion and spirituality. Nonetheless, recent polls such as those undertaken by the Pew Forum on Religious Life[1] have shown that the religious impulse is as strong as ever. With ninety-two percent of respondents indicating belief in God or a universal spirit, it is obvious

Yoga – Philosophy for Everyone: Bending Mind and Body, First Edition.
Edited by Liz Stillwaggon Swan.
© 2012 John Wiley & Sons, Inc. Published 2012 by John Wiley & Sons, Inc.

that people still value spiritual experience. But, as identification with traditional Western religions declines,[2] it is becoming clear that the spiritual needs of the United States, and other Western cultures, are changing.

According to *Yoga Journal*, as many as fifteen million people in the United States practice yoga. The past twenty years have seen a rapid rise in yoga's popularity, and in many major cities today there seems to be a yoga studio on every other block. What accounts for this sudden growth, and is it related to the changing religious landscape? What are people getting out of it? Is yoga a religion? After watching my yoga students, as well as my own practice, I've come to believe that the practice of yoga serves our everyday spiritual needs in a way few other spiritual practices are able to do. The rising popularity of yoga is an indicator of a shift toward a more eclectic and experiential spirituality.

Sweat, Stretch, and Practical Philosophy

Clearly, when students come to take class at my yoga studio, these considerations are not at the forefront of their minds. Most Western yoga classes, including mine, are pure Hatha yoga, a type of yoga that combines physical postures, called *asanas*, with such yogic touchstones as concentration, breath control, and efforts to create mental peace. Few yoga classes of this type include overtly religious or theistic elements, nor the ascetic practices described in many classical yogic texts. Yet many students feel that this type of Hatha yoga practice engages them spiritually. The practice has even led some to return to their religious roots, albeit with a more progressive interpretation of doctrine. In the West, yoga is usually associated with sticky mats, stretching, and relaxation. This physical practice, according to yogic philosophy, is only the tip of the iceberg. In India, the cradle of yoga, the physical discipline often takes a back seat to its more meditative, devotional, contemplative, or theistic forms.

Yoga holds wide appeal for Westerners, for reasons ranging from the obvious health benefits to subtler boons. Its non-competitive nature is a balm against the strain of our hyper-competitive world. In the calm and non-judgmental environment of a yoga studio, a vigorous practice of physical postures burns off our natural restlessness, allowing us to slow down and smell the roses, even if only for a few minutes before we return to our hectic lives. The spiritual teachings, which draw on the rich philosophical tradition of such works as the *Yoga Sutras* and the *Bhagavad Gita*, are interwoven into these physical classes. A common format, and one that I myself use, has come to be known as the '*dharma* talk.' This is a short, typically five-to-ten-minute talk on a specific aspect of the yoga philosophy. These talks often center on social responsibility, self-control, charity, compassion for the self and others, and a simplified life – ideas that can be quite appealing in our culture of continual grasping and rampant consumerism.

We usually associate such teachings with a religious service rather than a workout. Preachers and priests commonly exhort parishioners to 'do unto others ...' and so on, providing moral guidance and seeking to bolster values and morality. But, while the subject may be similar, the context of a yoga class is very different. Teachings on *karma* or non-violence are presented briefly and informally, in a way that is easy to absorb, even for those unfamiliar with the tradition. Typically, even if a yoga teacher is committed to a particular religious path, such as Buddhism, he will go out of his way not to push the path upon students. In my classes, I often qualify my statements by saying 'remember, these are just my ideas,' or 'this is the traditional view of the Vedanta philosophy.' The student is encouraged to make up her own mind.

These teachings are presented in such a way as to be practical, rather than merely metaphysical. This practical emphasis begins with the physical practice itself. The practice of *asana* coupled with yogic breathing can very quickly lead to a direct, if initially fleeting, experience of the peace promised by yoga. We feel firsthand the peaceful, relaxed state of mind that comes from a good yoga class. Compared to a hectic life, this sensation is very desirable, and opens the student to the deeper aspects of yoga. When we feel peace from our practice, we can look to the philosophy to keep that peace as we step off the mat. Often, I see first-timers in class staring blankly as I give my lesson of the day, not really understanding why they have to sit through all this talk. Their faces seem to say, 'I'm here to work my abs, not listen to you talk about truthfulness!' Quickly enough, though, they begin to feel the peace of the physical practice, and they become interested in the rest because they can see how it readily applies to their lives. A few classes later they're listening with rapt attention, and the philosophy begins to benefit them pragmatically.

A good example of the practicality of yoga philosophy is the first of the eight limbs of yoga. Yogis follow the *yamas*, or ethical restraints (non-violence, truthfulness, non-stealing, sexual chastity, and non-greed) less for any metaphysical reason, or due to the expectations of a particular divinity, than because they lead to personal and social peace. A yogi practices *satya*, or truthfulness, less because of a concern for what God might expect and more because they realize that lying and deception are usually more trouble than they're worth. Most of us can easily remember lying to our parents or teachers as a teenager, the constant worry of being caught in a lie, and how much work it was to keep our story straight. Obviously this does not lead to peace but to an anxious and distracted mind. This sort of practical technique, simply being truthful, leads to a more tranquil mind in anyone who tries it.

The sense of peace that can quickly arise in yoga classes, meditation, or philosophical study can be enough to initiate a spiritual life, or revitalize a flagging spiritual quest. It can lead people to live a more mindful life. One of my students, a not-particularly-observant Jewish woman with a classic New York accent, talks about how much the practice has calmed her. 'I'm very Zen now,' she likes to say with a boisterous laugh, 'I tell my friends, you *gotta* try yoga.' Loving how it makes her feel, she recently cancelled her gym membership to take yoga classes full time.

With yoga's steady growth in the West and its acceptance into the mainstream, we cannot dismiss it as a fad. With countless exercise regimes out there to choose from, and so many people choosing yoga, we can assume that there is a deeper need being met than a desire for rock-hard abs and open hamstrings. There is a change happening under the surface. Yoga students are looking for something deeper, and this need is emerging out of the roots of our shared history.

'I'm Spiritual, but not Religious.' What's the Difference?

A few years ago, I wrote a few articles for a New Age website. In writing this essay, I'm reminded of a bit of early correspondence with the editor of the website. Like any editor, this man had some very specific ideas about which articles to include and which to avoid. He explained that many of his readers were distrustful or had an aversion to traditional Western religions, but that Eastern religions were thought of as safer to discuss. For instance, I wasn't permitted to write about the *Spiritual Exercises of St. Ignatius of Loyola*, describing a Catholic method of meditation, but Zen gardens and Tibetan mandala meditation were fair game. For me, this raised a lot of questions. I wondered, what does this say about the religious culture of the United States?

It is always difficult to accurately see the web of ideas, preconceptions, and prejudices that create our mental outlook. We're just too close to see the whole picture. Religion is a big part of our paradigm, whether or not we're believers. Everyone who was raised in the West has a common religious inheritance that is broader than the specific religion we may have been born into. But, while this inheritance may be shared by all, it is continually evolving, like any aspect of a shared culture. Religion has never been an unchanging monolith of truth, nor have believers of the same sect ever held precisely the same beliefs. However, when we think of religion we tend to think of a set of dogmas that claims to capture some absolute and unchanging truth. Certainly it may seem that every preacher assumes this eternal and exclusive nature in doctrine, even when he disagrees with the preacher on the next pulpit over. We see this religious inheritance even in the more extreme atheists, who, in rejecting religious teachings absolutely, become the fundamentalists in the cult of reason. The force of history may be eroding this absolutism, but as of today it forms part of the ground of our religious understanding. Today, when we think about religion, we often think of the loudest of these absolutist voices, whether fighting against the teaching of evolution, preaching intolerance and bigotry, or even strapping explosives to their chests. These negative images have certainly contributed to the rejection of traditional religion, but they have not destroyed the religious impulse itself. This rejection drives many people to label themselves as 'spiritual' and not 'religious.' Is there a difference?

In everyday speech we tend to use to the words 'religion' and 'spirituality' interchangeably, but for this discussion the two ideas must be distinct. The word religion comes from the Latin *religare*, 'to bind together' – literally, we can say religion is what binds people together. It is natural then to include here a common set of values, shared myths, rituals, and holidays marking time or life stages, and other reference points held in common by a community. This is certainly the way religion was understood in many ancient cultures, where there was no distinction between the personal, political, and religious. Today we see remnants of this in the Jewish faith, which identifies itself as a religion, a culture, and even a distinct ethnicity. Spirituality comes from a different word, *spiritus*, 'of breath' or 'of the spirit,' from which we also derive the words 'inspire' and 'respiration.'

From this we'll say that religion is a culturally specific set of teachings and dogmas, claiming to explain both the nature of the world and what we should value in it, that unites a people or congregation, whereas

DAVID ROBLES

spirituality is the personal derivation of value and meaning, dependent on individual inspiration and revelation. As we shall see, although the yoga tradition originated in a culturally Hindu setting, it is entirely concerned with personal revelation rather than cultural norms. Yoga is then a spiritual practice, and does not serve the same function as a religion.

We can consider religion to be the agreed-upon norms of the group in regard to their spirituality. It is therefore only natural that all religions are inherently conservative; they must hold their common norms against the constancy of change. If those norms are absolutist (e.g., this is the 'one true way' and every other way is wrong), then these norms cannot be expected to change with the times, but must be eternal, unchanging truths. If X was true for the religious founder, no matter what has transpired since he walked the Earth, it must be true now. This is exactly the religious inheritance of the West as it comes down to us today from the Abrahamic tradition, which includes Judaism, Christianity, and Islam.

Distrust of authority and the ideal of personal liberty have also helped erode the prominence of traditional religions. As our world has become increasingly transparent, countless scandals have arisen that have undermined faith in traditional religion. These range from the personal failings and greed of charismatic preachers to the sexual abuse scandals of the Catholic Church. Many people flocked to Eastern Gurus over the course of the twentieth century, hoping that by trusting a new authority they might be in better hands. This hope was not always fulfilled, and accordingly the distrust of religious authority has grown. The result has not only changed the Western view of religion but also the yoga tradition itself, which in the West places far less emphasis on the importance of the Indian tradition of absolute surrender to the guru.

A 'Spiritual Science' is not just an Oxymoron

One of the biggest fault lines in traditional religion today is the apparent disconnection with mainstream secular views, in particular the acceptance of science and the scientific method. Over the past few centuries, the hegemony of the Western religious tradition has broken down, and, where once a person could find all the explanations he needed in the Bible, science now takes on much of this role. As the value of evidence and empirical experience eroded the value of faith, and the wonders of science outstripped the rare occurrence of miracles, people naturally began to question their articles of faith, especially those dealing with the physical world. The fruits of science, fabulous inventions able to be seen and felt directly, lent great authority to this increasing body of knowledge, and, as theories were expounded that were in direct conflict with the explanations of religious doctrine, a sense of intellectual dissonance grew. People began to demand similar results from religion, and traditional religion has had a hard time meeting this demand. We have begun to desire results in this life, rather than the next.

Reactions among the faithful to the influence of science have, historically, varied. We have seen attempts to use science to prove the existence of God, as well as the prosecution of scientists and free-thinkers. Today science has largely won the battle, usurping many of the traditional functions of religion. For many, religion no longer serves the function of explaining the origin and nature of the world, although it still provides a system of values for many. Part of the difficulty is that when we accept a partial explanation (say, treating the Bible's creation story as metaphor, but believing in Heaven), we open ourselves up to feelings of intellectual unease and spiritual doubt. This causes many to rely less on the comparative vagaries of religion, as science seems to rest on a more concrete foundation. Perhaps it does, as it is based on evidence. But, while it may explain the world physically, it cannot tell us what the world, or our lives, mean. This leaves many secular folks with a sense that something has been lost in the shuffle.

Most religions are based on the idea of revelation. Not your revelation, mind you, but someone else's. This is the history of all religions: someone (usually the founder or founders of the religion) had an experience, and taught others, most of whom did not have the same experience themselves. Swami Vivekananda, in his classic book *Raja Yoga*, puts it beautifully: 'if you go to the fountain-head of Christianity, you will find that it is based on experience. Christ said he saw God; the disciples said they felt God; and so forth.'[3] These teachers (Christ, the Buddha, and so on) try to teach others how to have the same experience, and create a system of practices or a philosophy derived from these experiences. These in turn become dogmas, and, when accepted by a community, become religions. No matter what the culture or religion, these teachings have one thing in common: they are all second hand.

This idea that all religions are based on experience is the foundation for the philosophy of yoga. According to the *Yoga Sutras* of Patañjali, only three sources of knowledge are acceptable: direct perception, logical inference, and verbal testimony from a trusted source (including scripture.) We know something most directly when we see it, say a fire burning somewhere. We may detect the existence of fire, even if we can't see it, by inferring its existence logically by the presence of smoke. Similarly, we may also come to learn of its presence by the verbal testimony of a trusted source, as in a friend coming to tell you that a house down the street is ablaze.

In classical texts such as the *Sutras*, the order in which items are listed is significant. Regarding the three sources of right knowledge, the first type, direct perception, is treated as the most important, and indeed the origin of the others. This is similar to the scientific method, where we observe a phenomenon and attempt to make logical inferences about it. In yoga, we find a spiritual system that is actually in harmony with the scientific method. In Western (and most Eastern) religions, this order is reversed, valuing the traditional testimony of scriptures and their interpretation (inference) above personal religious experience. Most spiritual or religious systems ask others to subscribe to their tenants based on faith, traditional cultural association, or merely on the strength of assertion and charisma. Even religious individuals may doubt the likelihood of miracles, visions, and divine manifestations happening today. Yoga, conversely, agrees with science that anything that has occurred in the past can potentially occur in the future, assuming that conditions are the same. If Ramakrishna could attain ultimate enlightenment while on Earth, so can anyone who lives in the same manner and follows the same practices.

In contrast to the pre-eminence of scripture in mainstream religion, yoga's stance is radical. Established religion is inherently conservative, assuming that, if the teachings are the absolute truth, there is little need for updating, refinement, or proof. Attempts to procure personal revelation and gnosis (spiritual knowledge) independent of the accepted teachings of the local authority have traditionally been discouraged, sometimes persecuted. Even today, some Islamic authorities as well as influential American Baptists have banned or discouraged yoga practice for related reasons. No wonder ancient yogis preferred to live in remote caves and huts.

An important aspect of the modern drift toward spirituality over religion surely is its philosophical harmony with, or at least lack of contradiction to, science, but cultural factors also play a part. The specifically American religious tradition is certainly informed by that much-touted American trait of rugged individualism and self-reliance – what we might call the 'pioneer spirit.' Americans are in love with the idea of progress, and, just as it has always been the American way to build a better mouse trap, we can see a quintessentially American attempt to build a better spirituality. Keeping all this in mind, we can see that we are beginning to demand a form of spirituality that is based on individual effort, distrustful of second-hand information (dogma) and authority, and desirous of direct perception of truth by the individual practitioner.

A Bull Market (or a Market of Bull)

The conflict between science and traditional absolutist theology is not just played out in the newspapers; it's in the Western subconscious as well. It is part of what defines the religious quest in our time. Add to this a dash of rugged American individualism, a pinch of increasing consumerism, and the exposure to pluralism resulting from freedom of religion, and we get an idea of where we are today. The result is a rather confused mish-mash of ideas and cultures, and everyone is set adrift on an ocean of ecclesiastic uncertainty.

Some people react to this uncertainty by diving deeply into fundamentalist religions. These offer an easily grasped, clear-cut absolutist mentality and a hard-headed certainty that can be all too comforting against the diversity and chaos of the modern world. Others look for the same sort of rock-hard certainty in a materialist philosophy, either avoiding the spiritual question entirely or rejecting it so absolutely as to become what I call 'fundamentalist atheists.' Still others, unable to surrender reason to an absolutist religion but feeling that science cannot provide all they are looking for, choose another path. The Who aptly labeled this type 'the seeker' in their song of the same title.

These 'seekers' know they want or need something that others find in traditional Western religions, but are driven to find it in different ways. Some of these convert outright to Eastern religions, but most find the associated cultural trappings too alien. More commonly, these seekers develop personal methods, creating a customized set of beliefs and practices unique to them. The basic law of economics is that, if there is a demand, someone will come along and try to supply what is needed. This deep spiritual hunger in the West, particularly the United States, has created a vast marketplace of products, ranging from the traditional to the outright bizarre. These include spiritual retreats, alternative healing

DAVID ROBLES

practices, meditation classes, baubles, clothing, and books (like the one you're reading). Of all of the incredible variety of traditions currently to be found in the spiritual marketplace of the United States, none is more popular than yoga. Its practicality, venerable history, and openness have helped it stand above the rest.

Any God You Like

Globalization and cultural tolerance also have parts to play in our changing spiritual needs. Our world is shrinking, and we have been confronted with a sometimes bewildering diversity of ideas from other cultures. Slowly, our society is evolving to accommodate this ideological mixing pot. A portion of the aforementioned Pew Forum survey showed that, in contradiction to the absolutist doctrines of their faiths, a majority of Americans (seventy percent) believe their own faith is not the only path to salvation, eternal life, or personal happiness. While this varies from sect to sect, in our day-to-day lives we are seeing it become less acceptable to hold exclusionary views. How can the traditional absolutist stance survive in such an environment? This increasing tolerance, as well as increasing exposure to the diversity of religious belief, seems to be softening the edges of absolutist religious belief, and it is becoming more common to hold views at variance with one's local priest. Belief in reincarnation and *karma* are just two examples that are becoming increasingly common among those who identify themselves as members of traditional Western faiths.

The yoga philosophy, while containing many theistic elements, is inherently inclusive. While the *Yoga Sutras*, one of the most important works on yoga philosophy, is certainly theistic, stressing the importance of 'surrender to the supreme being,' its author is careful not to specify which supreme deity he is talking about. Instead, he tends to use such terms as *ishta devata*, or 'one's chosen deity,' instead of specifying Shiva, Krishna, or any other. Meditations prescribed in the *Sutras* rank meditation on the divine as the most effective for achieving the goals of yoga, but Patañjali generously includes many other suggested objects of meditation. After listing many possibilities, he concludes by flinging the doors wide with a verse offering as an object 'anything one chooses that is elevating.'[4] Such broadness has certainly contributed to the fact that this philosophy, born from a very specifically Hindu setting two thousand years ago, is incredibly popular centuries later and worlds away. Today Buddhists, Christians, and even atheists draw inspiration and direction from it.

Countless people who have never read the *Yoga Sutras* are practicing the above verse without realizing it. People are taking charge of their own spiritual education and meditating, worshiping, or otherwise drawing inspiration from any and all traditions that strike their fancy. I know several yogis who have chosen to meditate on the symbols or gods of ancient Egypt, or other now-extinct religious traditions. Not every seeker goes quite this far, but most seem to have no problem mixing and matching doctrines, deities, and practices from any number of faiths. Yoga seems a snug fit for this sort of globalized eclecticism.

Into the Future

From this broad overview we can conclude that, although attitudes toward religion are evolving rapidly in the United States, and in the West more generally, Americans are not necessarily losing that mysterious instinct to pursue spiritual or religious lives. Instead, we are in the process of painfully evolving our sense of what we should expect from religion and spirituality, be it traditional or otherwise. Whatever forms this may take in the future, we can be sure that our religious outlook will continue to evolve, changing as society changes. Presently, we are beginning to require that our faith be open rather than absolute, be self-directed rather than dogmatic, and, whenever possible, be in harmony with scientific knowledge.

I believe we are moving in the direction of a more self-directed spirituality, one in which any individual can take charge of his own spirituality, draw inspiration and direction from a variety of traditions, and demand results that can be experienced directly in this life. As our needs develop in this direction, teachings and teachers will rise to meet the demand. Yoga, for the moment, is well suited to such evolving needs. Whether this relationship will intensify or whether the West's love for yoga will sour, only time will tell, but we can be sure that, if the influence of yoga wanes, another spiritual practice will rise to fill the need. Until then, we can expect to hear the sound of 'om' resonating across the United States and elsewhere in the West.

DAVID ROBLES

NOTES

1 PEW Forum on Religion and Public Life, 'US Religious Landscape Survey' (June 23, 2008, http://pewforum.org/US-Religious-Landscape-Survey-Resources.aspx).
2 CUNY, 'American Religious Identification Study, 2001 (http://www.gc.cuny.edu/faculty/research_studies/aris.pdf).
3 Swami Vivekananda, 'Raja yoga,' in *The Collected Works of Swami Vivekananda, Volume I* (Advaita Ashrama, Kolkata, 1989), p. 126.
4 *Yoga Sutras of Patanjali*, trans. Swami Satchidananda (Integral Yoga Publications, Buckingham, VA, 1999).

CHAPTER 4

MEN, SPORTS, AND YOGA

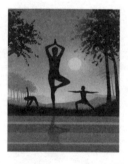

Do Real Men Do Yoga?

'Ask a regular guy if he does yoga, and he'll probably say, "I wouldn't be caught *dead* doing that crap – it's for girls,"' ex-professional wrestler Diamond Dallas Page writes in his fitness book *Yoga for Regular Guys*.[1] And you know what? He's right. Nearly eighty percent of yoga practitioners in the United States are female, according to a 2005 *Yoga Journal* survey. Yoga's gender gap is an oddity limited to the Western world; in India, yoga has actually been dominated by men since its inception.

'I can't think of a better place to meet women who are in great shape with great, flexible bodies than in the yoga studio,'[2] Page writes. Western yoga studios are frequented by women in tight clothing who contort themselves into positions with racy names such as 'downward facing dog' and 'supine goddess pose.' While this sounds like an intriguing set-up for many single, straight men, Western men have stayed away from yoga studios for the most part.

Yoga – Philosophy for Everyone: Bending Mind and Body, First Edition.
Edited by Liz Stillwaggon Swan.
© 2012 John Wiley & Sons, Inc. Published 2012 by John Wiley & Sons, Inc.

Every guy has at least one male friend who has tried yoga before and lived to tell the tale. For many guys, the tale isn't a pretty one. 'A world turned upside down – that's yoga for most of us men,' Andrew Tilin writes in *Yoga Journal*.[3] Co-ed yoga classes invert traditional gender politics in athletics, even if experience levels may have more to do with differences in skill than does gender.

Attempts to get men into the yoga studio have fallen flat. Take the 2003 book *Real Men Do Yoga*.[4] A great title, which unfortunately featured football star Eddie George on the cover ... shirtless and in his underwear. Even yoga enthusiast Page can't seem to go more than a few pages in his book without derogatorily mentioning the 'scrawny new-age girlie men'[5] that he sees in United States yoga studios.

Few men have been willing to come out of the yoga closet on the national stage and encourage fellow bearers of the Y-chromosome to take up this imported Eastern art. One of those men happens to be Major League baseball pitcher Barry Zito, who has practiced yoga since 1998. While he shares some of his regimen with teammates, he doesn't shove it down their throats. 'It's too foreign for them,' he tells *Yoga Journal*.[6] Part of the problem is that many Western men are obsessed with muscle size as an indicator of strength. Yoga challenges this belief. 'It's great that you can bust through a brick wall, but yoga takes a different kind of strength,'[7] personal trainer and yoga instructor Rebekah 'Bex' Borucki says.

Some men have found that participating in one-on-one yoga sessions – often outside the confines of gyms and studios – has given them the confidence to explore for themselves why yoga has been going strong for 5000 years. Barbara Purcell, a New York City-based yoga instructor (and co-author of this essay), has been teaching Vinyasa yoga to a number of men who prefer to practice in their home or office instead of the various yoga studios Manhattan has to offer. Private lessons ensure that these men, often quite successful in their lives and careers, can avoid exposing themselves to the embarrassing fear of failure that often plagues guys practicing in group-class settings.

The following three stories – each based on one of Barbara's male yoga students – illustrate a common theme among guys who have practiced in both one-on-one and group-class settings. (Names have been changed to protect the innocent. And inflexible. And out of shape.) It seems that, regardless of yoga's philosophical emphasis on non-judgment, universal connection, and ever-expanding self-awareness, there is still a competitive, ego-driven aspect to developing a personal yoga practice. Whether a student struggles to touch his toes during the first class or feels flustered when nearly toppling out of a headstand months, perhaps years, later, the push to perfect one's practice does exist. And it seems to be especially strong for men in Western cultures, where cultural gender bias holds that men are more competitive than women (whether this bias has any basis in fact is another issue). It appears that yogis struggle more than their yogini counterparts when the quest to perfect each pose is replaced with a greater self-realization that body and mind must reconcile their differences – at least while on the yoga mat.

Mark's Story: 'It was like Line Dancing for the First Time'

Mark is a forty-three-year-old senior director at one of New York's most reputable management consulting firms. As an active guy who has recently lost about 40 pounds, he enjoys golfing, downhill skiing, and the occasional jog. Mark came to Barbara for private yoga lessons after his massage therapist recommended yoga as a supplement to his weight loss plan. The assisted stretching during his massage therapy sessions always put him in a relaxed state, even before any healing hands were applied, making him open to learning more about the benefits of stretching and yoga in general.

In his initial one-on-one yoga sessions, Mark learned the various breathing techniques and explored the poses Barbara felt would work best for his body type and experience level. After three private sessions, he ventured off into the wild world of Manhattan yoga studios, where he settled into an 'open level' group class.

'I didn't know what the protocol would be the first time I went to class, which made the experience intimidating, even a little scary,' Mark reflects. He recalls seeing other first-timers there – especially men – who looked visibly shaken by the whole ordeal. While the class was not overtly competitive, the ego-based self-consciousness that he experienced was unavoidable. 'I didn't need to be better than the twenty-three-year-old women twisting themselves into pretzels, but, considering I couldn't even see my toes, I just didn't want to look stupid. It was like line dancing at a country western bar for the first time, not knowing the steps when everyone else does.' As Mark explains it, there were two types of yoga students in his class: those who could two-step and those who had two left feet.

As he became more comfortable with the environment, Mark gradually shed his competitive instincts. He continued to attend group classes while

BARBARA PURCELL AND ANDREW SHAFFER

also seeing Barbara for private lessons. Unlike the group classes, private lessons allowed him to pay more attention to his alignment, improve his technique, and work with specific sequences. After just a few sessions, Mark began to feel a major difference in his balance, flexibility, and core strength.

Perhaps most notably, he felt a significant improvement in his golf game. So good, in fact, that he began to tell his other golf buddies – men who were, for the most part, slightly older than him – about the benefits of yoga. To his surprise, they all admitted to also practicing in some capacity. One fellow golfer did not know that his stretches were ancient *asanas* (yoga poses), but rather thought they were designed for a better swing. Yoga is a 'dirty little secret' for most of these guys. The bottom line, according to Mark, is that anyone serious about his or her golf game could benefit from being equally religious about his or her yoga practice.

Although Mark himself has not experienced a 'spiritual awakening' from the various stretches and moves, he has tapped into the meditative quality of learning to link breath with movement while concentrating in various balances and poses. 'Even though group classes tend to talk more about the warm and fuzzy *chakra* stuff, I really appreciate how private lessons allow me to tap into the mind–body benefits. Like deeper concentration: that's something I can take with me off the yoga mat and onto the golf course or even to a business meeting.'

Perhaps the biggest surprise Mark has experienced from developing a personal yoga routine: 'I was breaking a serious sweat every time. It was a solid aerobic workout, just by standing still in certain poses,' he says.

Mark is a believer in the ancient Eastern art and openly shares it with golf enthusiasts as well as stressed-out colleagues and friends looking to improve healthy habits. Those initial feelings of self-consciousness in the group class setting have been replaced with a more relaxed attitude. 'Maybe it's an age thing, but after a while, you just can't care as much if the person on the mat next to you is better at touching his toes than you are.'

Carl's Story: 'Everyone Avoids the Front and Center in Class'

Carl is a fifty-one-year-old airline captain who works long shifts flying back and forth across the United States. The combination of many hours in the cockpit, the stress associated with flying, and the constant lugging of his heavy bags on and off planes all contributed to chronic tightness and upper spinal issues. A former avid hockey player, he is still extremely fit and works out by lifting weights regularly at the gym.

A few years ago, he decided to try a yoga class after his wife convinced him it would be a good way to manage his general tightness and neck/back discomfort. Reluctantly, Carl attended a 'basics' yoga class at his gym. The group was composed of about fifty adults, mostly female. Despite feeling out of his element, he maintains that the gender imbalance didn't bother him greatly.

Carl did not anticipate being so challenged, though, by the various poses and sequences. 'I really appreciated using my muscles in a different way that weightlifting didn't address; yoga offered a more complete work-out,' Carl says. 'I also missed the meditative quality that playing ice hockey once offered, so it was great to rediscover that same effect though yoga.'

Another aspect of hockey that Carl missed was competition. Yoga has also provided him with an adrenaline rush in this area, but not in the way he expected. 'It's not that I've ever felt that a yoga class was a competition, but I enjoy pushing myself and my own limits in order to improve.' After some gentle prodding, he admits yoga has also had a calming effect on him. 'I could see myself practicing yoga in one way or another for the rest of my life,' he says.

Carl prefers one-on-one lessons since a private instructor 'fine tunes the student's technique,' but, with changes in his work schedule and economic pressures, he's been more active with group classes at the gym. 'I do hope to get back to private lessons regularly in the near future,' he says. 'The attention to detail raises my awareness of each pose, which creates a much more challenging class.'

For now, Carl finds himself attending a weekly class filled with about fifty students, mainly middle-aged adults, who rarely talk to each other before or after the class. 'Most people are sort of living in their own bubbles,' he says, later explaining that many residents of his Westchester town are generally aloof. Does the large group, with its wide range of experience levels, create a sort of class hierarchy? Do well-versed yogis sit in the front of the room? 'No,' he says, laughing. 'Everyone avoids the front and center unless they have no choice.'

Ultimately, though, he feels that, being a bit older, he's not terribly concerned about what other people are thinking of his yoga moves; in fact, he appreciates being on a mat next to an advanced practitioner as he or she is 'a good source of info' in keeping his own practice in check.

Carl feels the single most important benefit of yoga has been an improvement in his spinal health. He doesn't share this with other colleagues – he said he hardly mentions it, though once in a while he'll encounter another pilot who practices. 'It really helps with the pain. I'm not necessarily advertising that to others, but I'm definitely not hiding it either.'

Jake's Story: 'The only Judging going on is in my Own Head'

Jake is a sixty-one-year-old oculoplastic (eye) surgeon who runs practices in both New York City and New Jersey. His work schedule is quite hectic and he has little time to relax other than on weekends, which he often fills with swimming, walking, and Sunday yoga classes. Despite (or because of?) his five am weekday wake-up calls and long hours in the operating room, Jake is a trim man with lots of energy. He performs a nightly stretching routine before going to bed, which has been helpful for much of his chronic tension and stiffness.

He enjoys the overall relaxation he feels after yoga practice. 'I never thought yoga could be so strenuous, but I was wrong on that front. It's proven to be my most physically challenging form of exercise,' he says, echoing the thoughts of many other men who have scoffed at the 'girl sport.'

Jake initially began his yoga practice through group classes at a local gym. Barbara has worked with him one-on-one intermittently through the years as a way to polish up his alignment and technique in preparation for group classes. Jake appreciates the attention to detail inherent in private lessons; teachers in group classes often overlook certain physical issues as a result of leading many students at once. 'Often, I don't know whether or not I'm doing the pose correctly in class, but private lessons offer clarity about each move. The constant adjustments and assisting in a one-on-one lesson made me realize just how much I was missing in the faster-paced group setting.'

Although Jake prefers the private lessons to group class, he's quite happy with what his gym offers. 'It's a nice mix of people; I'd say about thirty percent men.' Do these classes have a competitive edge or does he ever feel judged by the other participants? 'The only judging going on in that class is in my head, and about my own limits,' he says. While he is blessed with a good sense of physical self-awareness, there is no 'yoga perfect' – there is only yoga practice. This knowledge helps him keep his competitive instincts (and ego) in check.

Competing against their own Bodies (but is it More than a Workout?)

All three of Barbara's surveyed students feel that yoga has offered them many benefits. Yoga has been a positive supplement to their individual lifestyles, both as a relaxation technique and as a core strengthener. Still, what keeps them returning to it week after week isn't a higher level of enlightenment; instead, the men are addicted to yoga for the physical workout it offers.

Could it be said that men who take private yoga lessons are competing against their own bodies? It certainly seems that someone like Mark, determined to lose weight and get in shape, found that yoga forced him to face just how challenging these poses and core-strengthening sequences could be. Had he simply encountered the 'fuzzy *chakra* stuff' emphasized in certain yoga studios, would he have stuck with it long enough to experience its notable effects on his golf swing or would he have crossed it off his dance card altogether?

But men aren't the only ones who seek yoga for its physicality. Rebekah Borucki writes on her *Philadelphia Magazine* health and wellness blog:

> Although I'd heard great things about yoga from my friends and colleagues, the first time I tried it I felt the same skepticism about what it could possibly offer me that many guys still feel today. And, unfortunately, my first class confirmed my fears. It was in my local gym, there was new-age synthesizer music playing, and the class was filled entirely with women. I didn't break a sweat and I vowed never to go again.[8]

Borucki eventually found her niche at a different yoga studio in New York City. 'I went to five different classes before I found one I liked,' she says. 'If I'm not sweating my way through a routine, pounding every muscle into submission, then I'm not working out.' Every yoga studio and class offers a different experience, and Borucki feels that classes with less emphasis on spiritual components are better suited to men who are beginning their yoga journeys. Otherwise, they run the risk of being alienated by its energy-based, subtle body effects. Before they can head toward nirvana, they should probably experience the perks of lower back relief or stronger abs. Most guys she knows who share her attitude on working out simply 'need to know how awesome yoga can be.'

BARBARA PURCELL AND ANDREW SHAFFER

Diamond Dallas Page knows how awesome yoga can be. He turned his book, *Yoga For Regular Guys*, into a 'fitness system' called 'YRG.' As rocker Rob Zombie writes in the introduction to Page's book, 'If you're anything like me, you know that even the sound of the word *yoga* will get you a sarcastic roll of the eyeballs.' Page changed Zombie's mind. 'Hey, I figured if *this* guy thought yoga was a bad-ass workout, maybe – and I emphasize maybe – there might be something to this New Age voodoo,' Zombie writes. And did it work? 'After about fifteen minutes of trying not to laugh, I realize this ain't exactly what I thought it was. This is difficult … .'[9]

The physical demands of yoga are just one piece of the puzzle, but they're an important one. 'We need physical exercise to deconstruct the ego that we've built up,' Neal Pollack, author of *Stretch: The Unlikely Making of a Yoga Dude*, says.[10] But, he emphasizes, physical yoga is still only one branch on the yoga tree. Beyond the veneer of sweat and muscle pounding lies yoga's hidden trove of mental bounties. 'Yoga's internal rewards – everything from better focus to less stress – are the hardest for men to realize,' writes Andrew Tilin in *Yoga Journal*.[11] He cites men's competitively wired brains as a barrier to achieving intellectual or emotional results. Pollack concurs. 'Not only did I find it difficult to lose my ego, I had no clue it was what I was supposed to do,' he says.[12]

Competing against other People (perhaps the Real Competition is within Yourself)

'For men, physical activity – non-sexual physical activity – has always been closely associated with competition,' neuropsychiatrist Louann Brizendine tells *Yoga Journal*. 'Studies have shown that for the last 40 years.'[13] In order to gain traction with men, should yoga harness men's competitive instincts?

Some yogis, such as Bikram yoga instructor Luke Strandquist, are campaigning for *hatha* (physical) yoga to be accepted into the Olympic Games as a competitive sport. According to the *Telegraph*, participants would be judged on 'strength, flexibility, alignment, difficulty of the optional poses, overall demeanor and execution.' However, even yoga competitors realize that competitive yoga requires a different mindset. 'I realized that there was no point in comparing myself to the other competitors. The only thing I could do was show the judges what my body could do,' UK champion Matt Farci tells *The Daily Telegraph*.[14]

Even in a local yoga studio, 'you're constantly competing with yourself to stretch further, bend deeper, and eventually nail that pose,' writes Borucki.[15] The students that Barbara interviewed also agreed that the biggest form of competition came from within themselves, rather than from fellow students or the teacher.

Carl felt he showed good sense in arriving early enough to class to get the ideal spot: anywhere but the front and center of the room. Regardless of a student's experience level, practitioners hesitate to put themselves on display in a group setting, perhaps for fear of somehow embarrassing themselves in front of their fellow down-doggers. Men like Carl – already quite fit and flexible – may thrive in a one-on-one setting but feel less secure when introduced into a densely populated gym class of varying skill levels.

The message here is that guys need to be willing to give up competition with the limber woman next to them and focus on their own progress. Alpha male displays of dominance have no place in yoga studios. Letting go of the need to be one of the best (or at least not one of the worst) in class requires some serious retooling of the ego.

Competing against their Own Egos (Playing Nice with your Ego)

It's only natural that, when someone is told to 'obliterate their ego,' he or she gets defensive; first and foremost, the ego always seeks to protect itself. 'It's my ego,' writes Kristin, who blogs at *Namaste From Duluth*, 'Why would I want to remove this part of me any more than one of my limbs?'[16]

Ego is a dirty word in many yoga circles, but it's also an important part of what drives people into yoga studios in the first place. 'It's the ego that drives us (or at least me) to be so goal oriented,' writes Leah Castella on her *Yoga Journal* blog. 'I'm cursed (or blessed, depending on your perspective) with a strong desire to be good at things.'[17]

Jake also recognized the role of his own ego – both in one-on-one lessons and during group class. He seemed totally aware that the only obstruction to his practice was coming from his own head, which in turn freed him up enough to appreciate the importance of alignment and attention to detail within each pose. Rather than fret about what other people thought of his practice, his own internal judgment helped him to excel – both in the privacy of his own home and at the gym.

BARBARA PURCELL AND ANDREW SHAFFER

The Sanskrit word for ego is *ahamkara*, which means 'the I maker.' Instead of striving to obliterate the *ahamkara*, argues Sally Kempton in *Yoga Journal*, we need only keep it in check:

> A truly healthy ego would be one that did its job of creating necessary boundaries and kept us functioning as individuals. But rather than seeing itself as bounded by the personality, or identifying with its thoughts and opinions, this ego would know the real secret – that the 'me' who calls itself Jane or Charlie is just the tip of the iceberg of something loving and free that is living as 'me.' All that is. Greater than the greatest. Higher than the highest.[18]

'Whenever I climb I am followed by a dog called "ego,"' German philosopher Friedrich Nietzsche is often quoted as having said.[19] It's a tough dog to shake. Nevertheless, 'the guys coming to yoga have to be ready for the next level, be ready to let down their defenses,' Manhattan yoga instructor Michael Lechonczak tells *Yoga Journal*.[20]

The ultimate goal of all yoga is to achieve *dharma-megha samadi*, an enlightened state of mind beyond form or emptiness. 'The ego separates from the self and the practitioner realizes that he's powerless to control the vagaries of an endlessly shifting universe,' Pollack explains.[21]

This is, obviously, a very heady concept for yoga newbies. The good news for men is that getting to that next level doesn't mean they have to give up the things that make them who they are. 'Trying to live as ego-less as possible doesn't mean you can't play fantasy football or drink a beer,' Pollack says. 'It's just that you have a different attitude towards those things in your life.'[22]

So, it seems that yoga is an exercise in enhancing one's perspective – learning lessons on the mat and taking them forward in everyday life. And, if the ego is the main contender when increasing self-awareness, attaining greater universal connection, and getting a cute yoga butt, it seems that the process of unifying the mind and body is, in fact, a competitive sport after all.

NOTES

1   Diamond Dallas Page, *Yoga for Regular Guys: The Best Damn Workout on the Planet* (Philadelphia, PA: Quirk Books, 2005), p. 8.
2   Ibid, p. 14.
3   Andrew Tilin, 'Where are all the men?' *Yoga Journal* (March 2007), p. 192.

4   John Capouya, *Real Men Do Yoga: 21 Star Athletes Reveal their Secrets for Strength, Flexibility, and Peak Performance* (Deerfield Beach, FL: Health Communications, 2003).

5   Page, *Yoga for Regular Guys*, back cover.

6   Tilin, 'Where are all the men?' p. 128.

7   Rebekah Borucki, personal interview (2010).

8   Rebekah Borucki, 'Hot guys take yoga, not just in Philly,' *Be Well Philly* (blog post, October 7, 2010, http://blogs.phillymag.com/bewellphilly/2010/10/07/hot-guys-take-yoga-just-not-in-philly).

9   Page, *Yoga for Regular Guys*, p. 7.

10 Neal Pollack, personal interview (2010).

11 Tilin, 'Where are all the men?' p. 129.

12 Pollack, personal interview.

13 Tilin, 'Where are all the men?' p. 129.

14 Melissa Whitworth, 'Are you cool enough for competitive yoga?' *The Daily Telegraph* (June 7, 2010).

15 Borucki, 'Hot guys take yoga.'

16 Kristin, 'The philosophy of the ego,' *Namaste from Duluth* (blog post, February 15, 2008, http://namastefromduluth.blogspot.com/2008/02/philosophy-of-ego.html).

17 Leah Castella, 'Injured,' *Yoga Journal* (blog post, June 4, 2007, http://blogs.yogajournal.com/makeover/leah_castella).

18 Sally Kempton, 'Sophisticated ego,' *Yoga Journal* (March 2006), pp. 80–81.

19 While this quote is regularly attributed to Nietzsche in books and the public imagination, it does not actually appear in any of Nietzsche's published works.

20 Tilin, 'Where are all the men?' pp. 95–96.

21 Pollack, personal interview.

22 Ibid.

CHAPTER 5

STANDING ON YOUR HEAD, SEEING THINGS RIGHT SIDE UP

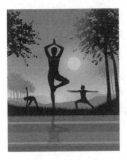

Yoga Theory

Yoga came into my life unexpectedly more than a quarter of a century ago, and I have been infatuated with it ever since. It has turned me upside down, bent me forwards and backwards. It has twisted me, and made me balance on my hands, arms, and elbows. It has taken me to extremes of exertion and relaxation. It has made me reflective, pensive, and inquisitive. It has developed my heart, brain, and courage. It has made me feel good about my accomplishments and humbled by my shortcomings – as well as humble about my accomplishments and good about my shortcomings. It has given me an experience of the range of the breath – from strong, full, and expansive, to fine, thin, and rarified. It has given me the experience of the floor of the pelvis releasing from the inner ears, the sensation of the palms softening with the relaxation of the thighs, and the resonance of different sounds in the back of my sternum.

But my infatuation is not unmixed: I have kept at arm's length the ancient Indian theories of humans and the world in whose terms the

Yoga – Philosophy for Everyone: Bending Mind and Body, First Edition.
Edited by Liz Stillwaggon Swan.
© 2012 John Wiley & Sons, Inc. Published 2012 by John Wiley & Sons, Inc.

practice of yoga is commonly described. For example, I am enthralled by deep backbends, but not by the claim that backbends stimulate *chakras*. I get absorbed in nuances of the breath, but I balk at the idea that the breath is connected with *prana*. I spend a lot of time in sitting postures, but I shrug when it is said that I am thereby awakening *kundalini* energy stored near the base of the spine.

Chakras, *prana*, and *kundalini* are just a few concepts from ancient Indian theories used to describe yoga. Let me briefly explain these, and a few other concepts, from these ancient theories. *Chakras* are centers of energy aligned along the spine from the floor of the pelvis to the crown of the head. *Kundalini* is a latent force stored at the base of the spine that can be awakened by the touch of a guru, or certain yogic practices. It then moves through the *chakras*, and, upon reaching the *chakra* at the crown of the head, the result is union of the limited self with the universal self. *Prana* is a vital force, closely linked to the breath. It pervades a human being, and is connected with other fundamental forces in the universe. A human being is enveloped by several *koshas*. These are sheaths or coverings, sometimes referred to as subtle bodies. They include *annamaya kosha* (related to food and the gross, or physical, body), *pranamaya kosha* (related to *prana* and other vital airs), *vijnanamaya kosha* (the sheath of the intellect), and *anandamaya kosha* (the sheath of bliss). Aspects of yoga are related to a spiritual dimension of the world – sometimes to God or gods; a soul that migrates from life to life; or an aspect of human nature, *purusa*, that transcends the natural order, an eternal consciousness or something like that. (For more details regarding ancient theories of yoga, an interested reader may look at classic texts, such as Patañjali's *Yoga Sutras*, written between 100 BCE and 500 CE; the *Samkhya Karika*, a central text of the Samkhya school of Indian philosophy, composed by Isvara Krishna *circa* 200 CE; and the *Hatha Yoga Pradipika* by Svatmarama, dating from the fifteenth century.)

Again, while I love having my body, mind, and breath bent and stretched, invigorated and soothed by the practice of yoga, I have doubts about the use of ancient Indian theories to describe yoga. Here is my concern: ancient theories of chemistry or physics or diseases are no longer taken to give literally true descriptions of things. They were discarded long ago in favor of more accurate and comprehensive theories in the sciences. Shouldn't we have the same attitude toward the ancient Indian theories used to describe yoga? Why do so many practitioners and teachers of yoga continue to use terms drawn from those ancient theories? Is the acceptance of such theories an example of modern irrationalism? Wouldn't it be more accurate and useful to think about yoga in terms of more modern theories of humans and the world?

Of course, the doubts I have expressed assume that contemporary theories in the sciences are more accurate than ancient Indian theories used to describe yoga, and this may be controversial. In this essay, I want to take a look at this assumption, and consider whether it can be reasonable to believe ancient Indian theories of yoga. Specifically, the question is this. In light of the evidence available to a moderately well-educated Westerner in the early twenty-first century, such as myself, can it be reasonable to believe that ancient Indian theories of yoga are true? (Hereafter, I refer to these theories as 'yoga theory.')

Here is how I proceed with this question. I begin with a fundamental objection to belief in yoga theory, which I call 'the standard objection.' It asserts that it is not reasonable to believe yoga theory because it has been superseded by superior theories in the sciences. I then spend much of the essay looking at a number of answers to this objection in defense of belief in yoga theory. The first few answers I look at are popular but clearly faulty. Another answer I look at appeals to testimony. The answer claims that, because of the crucial role of testimony in our beliefs about the world, it can be reasonable for many people to believe yoga theory even if it has been superseded by developments in science. I endorse this answer, but with an important qualification: the answer only applies to people with limited understanding of science. Toward the end of the essay, I outline several strategies for defending yoga theory that are not subject to this limitation. They include influential and controversial views about revelation and relativism, as well as the view that elements of yoga theory are preserved in the best current scientific theories, and so are as reasonable to believe as those theories themselves. I conclude the essay by considering how a serious practitioner of yoga should respond if the news is all bad – that is, if it turns out that it is not reasonable to believe any part of yoga theory.

Let me add that what I call 'yoga theory' includes theories about many aspects of the world – the inanimate physical universe, human anatomy and physiology, the mind, the self, moral aspects of the universe, and God. The reader may wonder to which of these theories my discussion applies. The answer is that most of my points are very general, and do not depend on which particular subject is at issue. When it does make a difference, I let the reader know.

Against Yoga Theory: A Standard Objection

In this section, I explain a fundamental objection to accepting yoga theory. I call it 'the standard objection.' The objection claims that the most dependable sources of knowledge about the world are found in the sciences. Theories in the sciences are based on observation, controlled experiments, and methods of hypothesis-testing, and for this reason they are more credible than theories based on tradition, ancient texts, enlightened masters, superstition, mystical insight, and such things. Galileo's views about motion and Copernicus' views about the revolution of the Earth around the sun, based on observation and hypothesis-testing, were more credible than the views of the church in their time, which were based on sacred tradition; and the views of modern geology and astronomy regarding the age of the Earth are more credible than the view that the Earth is approximately 6000 years old, which many people believe on the authority of the Bible. (Of course, the foregoing assumptions about science can be challenged, and later in the essay I briefly consider a few such challenges. Readers interested in such issues may consult literature on Hume's 'problem of induction' as a starting point for further investigation.)

Well, what does this have to do with yoga theory? With the growth of science, yoga theory, like other ancient theories, has been replaced by superior theories. Theories in contemporary natural science – for example in biology, anatomy, physiology, chemistry, physics, and neuroscience – are better instruments for prediction and explanation than the theories they have replaced. The standard objection says that we should reject much of yoga theory just as we reject other early theories of the world. We don't accept geocentric theories of the universe because heliocentric theories are better scientific theories. Early biologists believed in spontaneous generation of organisms. Some early theorists believed there were ultimately just five elements (earth, air, fire, water, and ether), and some thought that there is a substance called 'phlogiston' involved in combustion. Given the progress of science, it is unreasonable for contemporary educated people to accept early theories like these; and, for the same reason, it may be unreasonable for them to accept yoga theory.

Of course, early theories may have been reasonable for people in ancient times given the evidence they had available. But, relative to contemporary science, it is simply not reasonable to believe early theories like these.

STEVE JACOBSON

The vocabulary of yoga theory can lend an air of mystery and depth to yoga, but we should recognize yoga theory for what it is – an interesting, exotic, but very likely false view of humans and the world.

Some Inadequate Responses to the Standard Objection

Some people point out that contemporary science is fallible. Surely it could turn out that current theories in science are wrong and yoga theory is right. I grant this. But many things are possible that we have no reason to believe. Take, for example, the belief that the total number of pine needles in the state of Maine in the year 1911 was an even number. Possible? Yes. Is there evidence to believe it? Clearly not. Similarly, yoga theory is possibly true. But that does not mean that there is evidence that makes it reasonable to believe.

Another answer I have often heard is that yoga theory and contemporary scientific theories are just different ways of thinking about the world. That we favor one (the scientific one) is just a prejudice reinforced by society. This answer does not address the issue. Of course, some beliefs are reinforced by society. Whether reinforced by society or not, some theories are better than others: they provide better predictions and explanations of natural phenomena. Whether reinforced by society or not, the theory that the Earth is roughly spherical is better supported by observation and experiment than the theory that the Earth is flat; and some theories about the causes of the bubonic plague are better supported than others.

Some people support portions of yoga theory by appeal to extraordinary experiences they have had during yoga practice. There are reports of out-of-body experiences, extraordinary states of consciousness, a feeling of the heart *chakra* opening, and so on. In the face of such claims, it is important to be clear about what is at issue. The issue is not whether people have had powerful and unusual experiences. That is admitted. The issue is: what is their significance? For example, people can have moving experiences they describe as the heart *chakra* opening, like some people can have spooky experiences they describe as hearing and seeing ghosts. This does not necessarily make it reasonable to believe that there are either ghosts or heart *chakras*. The most sensible story seems to be that extraordinary experiences in yoga are the result of momentary alterations in brain chemistry and the nervous system produced by yogic practices, just as extraordinary experiences can be the result of altering brain chemistry by means of alcohol and other drugs.

I do not rule out the possibility that some very extraordinary experiences can make it reasonable to accept some portions of yoga theory that conflict with science. But I think such experiences are rare; and I think this card is likely to be overplayed by many people who would reject science on the basis of experiences they personally have had, when their claims would be rightly written off as resulting from excessive enthusiasm, gullibility, naïveté, superstition, or some other failure of critical judgment.

The Standard Objection and Testimony

I believe that it can be reasonable for many people to accept yoga theory, even if there is strong scientific evidence to the contrary; and I believe that no special experiences are required. My view begins with the idea that different people may hold the same belief for different reasons. Consider Charlie and Claire. Both believe that $e=mc^2$, but on very different grounds. Charlie is a very amiable regular at a local coffee shop. He is, well, dumb. He has had little schooling, and he is extremely gullible. One night a group of physics students tell Charlie that $e=mc^2$. Hearing it from the students, who are his coffee shop friends, Charlie comes to believe that $e=mc^2$. Had they said that $e=mc^3$, or that $e=mc^4$, Charlie would have believed that instead. Moreover, asked why we should believe that $e=mc^2$, Charlie has nothing to say – not because he is bashful: he simply has no idea what sort of evidence supports the belief beyond the fact that his friends told him that $e=mc^2$. Compare Charlie with Claire, a research physicist at the Institute for Advanced Studies at Princeton. The grounds for her belief are very different from Charlie's. Asked to justify the belief that $e=mc^2$, she knows the supporting evidence and experiments. She has conducted many of the experiments herself. She can explain why it would be a mistake to believe that $e=mc^3$ rather than $e=mc^2$. She can describe experimental outcomes that would make it reasonable to question or reject the belief.

Charlie and Claire are just two examples of people holding the same belief on different grounds. Take the belief that five-year-old Sam stole the cookies. Some, for example his little sister, may believe it only because they want it to be true. Some may believe it because they saw him do it. Some may believe it, not because they saw him do it, but because

STEVE JACOBSON

they know his personality and know that he had the opportunity to steal the cookies. Still others may believe it on testimony, having heard Sam's friends talk about Sam's daring daylight raid on the cookie jar.

As testimony is important to my view, let me say a bit more about it. Beliefs based on testimony depend on what we have read or been told. For example, we may have evidence that the defendant was at the church social, not because we saw her, but because the choir director told us that he spoke with her. We rely on testimony for beliefs about history (e.g., Caesar, the holocaust, the Boxer rebellion, and so on) and for beliefs about matters requiring expertise we lack. My belief about the problem with my car is based on what a mechanic tells me; and my beliefs about the Big Bang theory are based on the writings of astrophysicists.

In light of these points, let me explain how it can be reasonable for many people to believe yoga theory. Most contemporary people are not Charlie: they are smarter and have more education. But they are not Claire either. Observation and the methods of hypothesis-testing are supposed to be what confer scientific status on beliefs, but they play little or no role in the way in which many contemporary educated people accept the scientific picture of the world. For people like Claire, beliefs in scientific theories have genuinely scientific grounds, and for that reason their scientific beliefs have an appropriately high degree of credibility. But, for many contemporary people, beliefs in scientific theories have non-scientific grounds, such as the testimony of texts and teachers; and, for that reason, their beliefs have a lower degree of credibility – for example, the credibility of beliefs based on testimony, or, in worse cases, the credibility of beliefs based on bias or prejudice. Further, different non-scientific grounds for beliefs can confer different degrees of credibility.

Here are some examples. Relatively weak grounds for belief would be the way in which a child depends on the testimony of his or her parents, or a student depends on the testimony of a teacher. Somewhat stronger grounds would be testimony from a constellation of authorities – for example, clergy, teachers, elders, and parents. Still stronger grounds for belief would be critical reliance on authorities. Depending on what is at stake, people scrutinize sources of testimony more or less carefully: they are especially critical when sources disagree about matters of importance. People ask and answer questions such as these: Are the sources generally reliable? Do they have appropriate competence? Are they being sincere? Is there a conflict of interest or an ulterior motive?

How does all this apply to the question of the credibility of yoga theory versus the credibility of science? The point is that the strength of the grounds a person has for a scientific belief can fall anywhere on a continuum between Charlie and Claire. The same is true about the grounds a person has for believing doctrines of yoga theory. The issue of the rationality of belief in yoga theory comes down to the question of comparing the grounds a person has for believing a scientific theory with their grounds for believing yoga theory. It is possible that some people have relatively weak grounds for belief in science, for example bias or prejudice, and relatively strong grounds for belief in yoga theory, for example critical reliance on testimony. For such people, it would be reasonable to believe doctrines of yoga theory, even if those doctrines conflict with the best-supported scientific theories of the world.

Suppose you point out that I've only shown that accepting yoga theory over science can be reasonable at relatively low levels of rationality – for example, in the way that critical acceptance of testimony is more credible than bias, prejudice, or lower levels of testimony. I agree. I look at the higher end of the scale of rational belief below. Even so, for many people, it does not take very strong grounds to make yoga theory more credible than science. One reason is widespread scientific illiteracy: many people have very little understanding of contemporary scientific theories or the nature of science in general. Another reason is the highly specialized nature of science. It takes a great deal of effort and training to gain even a moderate degree of expertise in ever-narrowing branches of scientific knowledge. For example, one is not an expert in chemistry but inorganic chemistry, and not the entire sweep of inorganic chemistry but a very narrow branch. For this reason, science and science-based disciplines are often misrepresented in common beliefs of the public. For example, in weighing the credibility of a Western doctor's diagnosis and proposed treatment, one may be overly influenced by partial evidence, for example an awareness of the influences of the pharmaceutical corporations on the practices of medical doctors. Or, in reflecting on the merits of evolution theory, one may be influenced by authorities who wrongly discredit some of the methods involved in its explanation, such as carbon dating.

Putting together some of these points, we get a sobering picture. Suppose that science is the most reliable basis for forming beliefs about the world. Suppose that, in a society of freedom of thought and expression, the shopping malls of ideas display lots of options for belief – genuine scientific theories along with lots of counterfeits. Suppose that ignorance and misinformation about science are widespread – and that scientific investigation is conducted by an elite intellectual class, relying on methods of observation and hypothesis-testing largely unavailable to most members of society. Given the bases for belief many contemporary people rely on – for example weaker or stronger testimonial grounds – it is not surprising that many people have reasonable beliefs that conflict with the best-supported current theories in science, including, perhaps, belief in yoga theory.

Higher Up the Scale

What about higher up the scale of rational belief? Can yoga theory be reasonable for someone who has strong scientific grounds for scientific theories rather than, say, testimonial grounds? In this section, I propose various ways in which this can be true, though let me emphasize that whether any of the proposals I make are cogent requires a more in-depth investigation than I can undertake here.

Some people may claim that there are grounds in support of yoga theory that are stronger than optimal scientific grounds. In mystical traditions, there is the idea that by grace some people are granted a 'divine vision.' Similarly, there are alleged to be infallible sources of testimony that give beliefs more credibility than science. In Indian traditions, some schools assign this status to the Vedas; in the West, some assign this status to the Bible. Another view is that standards of rational belief are relative to cultures or traditions. Standards of scientific cultures are tied to methods of observation, induction, and hypothesis-testing. But one may claim that there are different standards of rationality in different cultures, and that, even if yoga theory is rejected by contemporary science, it can be perfectly rational to believe relative to the standards of, say, a traditional religious culture of which a contemporary person is a member.

Here is another possibility. Some doctrines of yoga theory may pertain to immaterial aspects of the mind or the self, beyond the reach of scientific theories of the natural world. Dualisms such as these are often part of religious belief, and based on faith or sacred texts. However, there is a tradition in philosophy going back at least to Descartes of attempting to establish doctrines such as these on rational grounds. There are arguments for such views based on reasoning about introspective features of the mind. On grounds such as these, one may try to establish that there is an eternal witness not causally involved in the world, or, more modestly, that there are subjective features of experience that are beyond the scope of the best naturalistic theories of the mind.

Moreover, some assumptions of yoga theory may be defended on the grounds that they are preserved in the best current scientific theories, and so are as reasonable to believe as those theories themselves. One such possibility draws from reflections about the history of science. In the early stages of inquiry, people theorized about such things as dogs, trees, stars, and atoms, and, with continued empirical inquiry and the growth of science, they developed better theories about these same things – better because they add information not contained in earlier theories, and better because they correct errors in earlier theories. On this view, it can be reasonable to think that there are such things as, say, *chakras* or *nadis*, even if it is not reasonable to share all or even many of the beliefs about them that are part of yoga theory. One may claim that the development of science has improved our understanding of these things, just as it has improved our understanding of many other things – the sun, the stars, space, time, and so on. Words such as '*nadis*' and '*chakras*' do not appear in the vocabulary of contemporary science, but contemporary science may have other words for the same things – just as the word 'water' does not appear in the vocabulary of chemistry, but chemistry has another term, 'H_2O,' for the same thing. In this way, modern science may agree with yoga theory that there are *nadis* or *chakras* (for example), even if it uses different words to talk about them and rejects many, if not all, of the views about them that are part of ancient yoga theory.

I have suggested how contemporary science may include elements of yoga theory. What if portions of yoga theory conflict with our best current scientific theories? Is it ever reasonable in such cases to accept yoga theory over science – without appeal to, for example, relativism or alleged infallible sources of testimony such as the Bible or Vedas? I believe so. Consider the following scenario. Bill studies under a highly reputed teacher of yoga from a lineage of practitioners dating back to antiquity. Bill's teacher, along with other members of the lineage, espouses a yoga theory that includes rich and detailed descriptions of conscious mental states experienced in different stages of yoga. Bill's teacher is a reliable source of testimonial evidence – modest in judgment; sincere; possessed of a mature, critical nature; and virtuous in other relevant ways. In the course of Bill's decades of study, the teacher has a good track record of predicting the new experiences he will have and the obstacles he will face. Moreover, Bill's teacher takes part in psychological studies on the physical foundations of the mental. In the course of these studies, Bill's teacher repeatedly reports experiencing different states of consciousness

STEVE JACOBSON

described by yoga theory, but the best current physical theories and instrumentation are unable to show any relevant physical difference when Bill's teacher reports being in one state or another. Suppose the same result is replicated many times by Bill's teacher and others in the lineage. Our best scientific theories tell us that there is no difference between the states of mind they report, whereas the evidence from Bill's teacher, and the others in the lineage, tells us there is a difference. In some such cases of disagreement, it seems reasonable to accept yoga theory over the best current science.

Conclusion

What if the news is all bad? What if it turns out that, at the higher end of the scale of reasonable belief, none of the foregoing considerations in favor of yoga theory pan out, and it is unreasonable for people with a good grasp of contemporary science to believe any part of yoga theory? What would be left of yoga? How should such serious practitioners respond? Should they retreat to dogmatism or unreason? I think not. My view is that abandoning yoga theory would no more diminish the practice of yoga than abandoning ancient theories of music would diminish the practice of music. Both practices are rich and rewarding, aside from whether ancient theories about them are right or wrong. Yoga, like music, would remain a fascinating, sometimes profound, path for exploring human nature. What would be left is yoga with fewer illusions.

PART 2

THE *ASANAS*: YOGA AND THE BODY

CHAPTER 6

HELP! MY PHILOSOPHY TEACHER MADE ME TOUCH MY TOES!

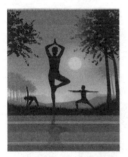

Imagine twenty students in a philosophy class, spread out on the floor like the spokes of a wheel. Their heads are in the center, and their teacher is guiding them to bring their attention to their bodies, from their feet, which form the wheel's circumference, to their heads, which form its hub. Finally they bring their awareness beyond their heads to the wheel's common center. What could they learn down there about the relationship between the universal and the particular, the collective and the individual, the whole and its parts?

Envision twenty students in a philosophy class, eyes closed, sitting tall, taking notice of the different sensations in the fronts and backs of their bodies, and thereby learning about their engagement with the world, with each other, and with themselves. Picture twenty students laughing hysterically as they fall out of tree pose the moment they close their eyes because their minds did not offer them a stable point of focus to help them maintain their balance. What could this teach them about the chaotic nature of our everyday minds? Later in the semester, imagine their surprise when they learn that, through their regular yoga practice, their minds have become sufficiently less chaotic so that they can, in fact,

Yoga – Philosophy for Everyone: Bending Mind and Body, First Edition.
Edited by Liz Stillwaggon Swan.
© 2012 John Wiley & Sons, Inc. Published 2012 by John Wiley & Sons, Inc.

maintain tree pose, even when they close their eyes. How much, and how deeply, could students learn in these ways about the nature of their minds, their bodies, and, indeed, all of philosophy's perennial questions?

In this essay, I'd like to share some of the ways I've been introducing yoga to my philosophy students these past few years in the hopes of inspiring other philosophy teachers to consider ways to teach yoga in their philosophy classes. Though my focus is on teaching, anyone interested in the intersection of philosophy and yoga should find something of interest here. I begin with some experiential exercises intended to introduce students to yoga's most fundamental philosophical concepts. I then explore ways of teaching two of Patañjali's famous eight limbs of yoga – *asana* (physical poses) and *pratyahara* (sense withdrawal). I conclude my exploration of the first, *asana*, by wondering what yoga's *asana* practices could bring to Western philosophy, asking, for instance, how our reflections on western philosophy's classic dilemmas might be aided were the philosopher to try reflecting while maintaining an appropriate yoga pose. I conclude my exploration of the second, *pratyahara*, by wondering, alternatively, what western philosophy might be able to bring yoga.

The Three Wheels Exercise

> If a beggar who thinks he is a king is mad, a king who thinks he is a king is no less so. (Jacques Lacan)

In this exercise, we create three wheels: two with pen and paper, one with our bodies. The first teaches that we have a true self; that is to say, an essential identity that can be distinguished from inessential, peripheral identities. This is not an especially foreign concept to students. The second wheel is more foreign: it introduces the central yogic teaching that the true self (what the teachings call *Atman*) is God (what the teachings call *Brahman*), or the essence of all reality. And, because we're always skeptical of foreign ideas, the third wheel attempts to engage that lesson through a more direct experience, bypassing the skeptical intellect. It is here that we make our first foray into yoga, when students get out of their chairs and, in this case, lay down on the ground...

To prepare for the first wheel, we discuss the various roles we each play in our lives: student, sister, son, worker, and so on. We then wonder what, if anything, holds them all together, making each of us one coherent person. I compare the roles to masks, our true selves to mask-wearers, and yoga to the project of removing all of the masks. To begin, each student writes ten 'I am' statements on a piece of paper (I am a student, I am a daughter...) and reads them aloud to the class. I explain that, since Aristotle, logicians have broken judgments down into their component parts: the subject (in this case 'I'); the copula, or conjugation of the verb 'to be' (in this case 'am'); and the predicate (in this case, 'daughter,' 'student'...). I then ask the students whether they would still be who they were if any of the words following each 'I am' (the predicates) ceased to apply to them. They eventually all usually agree that they would still be who they were and I argue that in a sense, then, the initial statements were actually untrue: the 'I' cannot be identified with the various predicates since it would continue to exist in the absence of any of the predicates. I am not, for example, a teacher; teacher is just an (inessential) mask that the (essential) I is wearing for a while.

To dramatize the point, I then ask the students to insert a 'not' after the ten 'I am's (I am *not* a student, I am *not* a daughter...) and then to read *that* list out loud to the class. I ask them to reflect on how it felt to read the list in this way, relating those feelings to the classical philosophical duality of the essential and inessential, and the quest for the true, essential self. In the experience of reading the list of negative judgments, I am essentially asking them to detach themselves from the predicates with which they normally strongly identify, and in this sense they have already entered the core of yoga by exploring *detachment*, in many ways yoga's most central concept.

Now the students draw their first wheel, consisting of a large circle (rim) with a smaller one in the center (hub) and ten lines (spokes) connecting the two. In the hub they write 'I am' and on each of the spokes they write one of the identities from the ten statements.

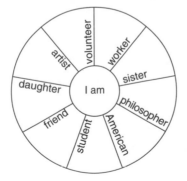

FIGURE 6.1   Wheel diagram by Josh Miller.

Next, they draw a second wheel. This time, each spoke is a different person. Though it will likely make little sense to them at first, I ask them to write 'I am' in the hub once more. This wheel is a bit more complex. For instance, Becky's journey from her inessential identities to her essential self is represented by her spoke. The journey is from the outermost point of the spoke, where it meets up with the circumference of the wheel, to the innermost point of the spoke, where it meets the hub of the wheel. To the extent that Becky identifies herself with her inessential identities, such as 'student,' she exists toward the outer circumference of the wheel. On the contrary, to the extent that she identifies herself with her true self, she exists toward the inner hub of the wheel. The same is true of me (Ken) – to the extent that I identify myself as a teacher, I exist on my spoke toward the outer circumference of the wheel. If Becky identifies herself as a student and I identify myself as a teacher, we are separate from one another, both on the wheel diagram and in our lives. But, if I identify myself with my true self and Becky does with her own self, then we both identify with the wheel's center, and we are no longer separated. We have, in the famous words of the Shvetashvatara Upanishad, awoken 'from this dream of separateness.'

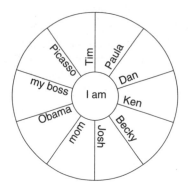

FIGURE 6.2   Wheel diagram by Josh Miller.

Thus, the intent of the wheel here is to illustrate the challenging yogic teaching that the true self of each individual is the same – that we all have, or better *are*, the same, universal self. We then turn to the Chandogya Upanishad, wherein the sage Uddalaka teaches his son that his essence is at once the essence not only of all other people but of all beings, from the fruit of the banyan tree to the rivers that flow into the sea: 'Believe me, my son, an invisible and subtle essence is the Spirit of the whole universe. That is Reality. That is Atman. Thou Art That.' I argue that the journey toward that truth, toward the true, universal self, is an excellent definition of yoga.

Now we'll turn to the really exciting part: the third wheel. This one requires the students to get up from their desks, and, in fact, to move those desks to the wall to create a clearing in the center of the room large enough for each student to lay on the ground so that they may form a wheel. Each student's body will constitute one of its spokes, their feet forming the rim and their heads forming the hub, which should be about four feet in diameter.

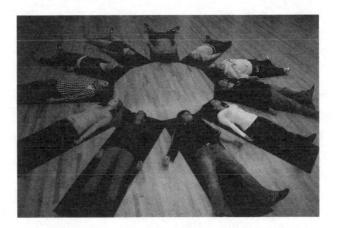

FIGURE 6.3   Reprinted with permission from Luis Vazquez.

I ask them to close their eyes and take a few deep breaths and then I guide them through a toe-to-head 'body scan,' asking them to bring their awareness from their toes, slowly on up to the crown of their heads, and then, finally, two feet beyond the crown of their heads to the wheel's center.

Once they have breathed a few breaths there, I tell them that all of their individual awarenesses are on the same point in the room. Indeed, if the hub is four feet in diameter, then two feet away from the crown of everyone's head is the center of the wheel. After one or two minutes, I ask them to follow their awareness back to the crown of their heads, then in a straight line down to their hearts, and then to let it rest there for a while as well. I note that a new circle, a circle within the circle, has been formed now, passing through each student's heart. Finally, I ask them to keep their eyes closed and come to a sitting posture, facing, and bringing their attention to, the center of the wheel. Soon they'll open their eyes, keeping their gaze on the room's center, then on each other, and, finally, they'll just relax.

In the ensuing discussion, the largest issues of philosophy, both Western and Eastern, will inevitably form themselves: the one and the many, the individual and the collective, the essential and the inessential, the universal and the particular, the body and the mind, the subject and the object, the I and the non-I, consciousness and existence... Indeed, the entire exercise is well suited to the first lesson of an introductory philosophy class since it doesn't presuppose any philosophical knowledge and ends with an experience out of which the basic problems of philosophy naturally emanate from the students themselves. And, at the very least, it gets their attention!

Teaching *Asana* in a Philosophy Class

A fun way to begin is with the speculation that the word 'yogi' initially referred to wild horse tamers. In yoga, the wild horses represent our minds. I elaborate with another horse–mind metaphor. A stranger approaches on a horse and is asked where he is headed. He replies: 'I don't know, ask the horse!' The horse is our mind and, without yoga, we are led where it takes us with little control over our destiny; that is to say, with little freedom. To experience the wildness of the mind, I simply ask the students to imagine an apple for a minute and then reflect on how difficult it was – how the mind, as we say, 'wandered.'

Just as the wheel exercise bids us to dis-identify with our masks, here we dis-identify with our minds. But then, if we're not our minds, who are we? The true self. Indeed, one stark contrast between Western philosophy and yoga is that, while Western philosophy tended to identify the true self with the mind, yoga does not – I am, after all, the horse rider, not the horse! – and bids us to take a distance from our minds and witness its workings. Otherwise put, whereas in Western philosophy we are defined by the duality of mind and body, in yoga there are always three terms: mind, body, and the true self, which is neither mind nor body nor a synthesis of both. But what is it, then? It is a witness who watches and is non-desirously, non-judgmentally, and non-conceptually present to the mind's many fluctuations.

Turning to Patañjali's *Yoga Sutras*, we find *yoga chitta vritti nirodha* ('Yoga is the cessation of the fluctuations of the mind'). Students are easily intrigued by the prospect of gaining some control over their wandering minds and are inspired to learn that having difficulty focusing is such an ancient problem. I ask, 'When we talk about attention deficit disorder, for what is it we don't have sufficient attention?' Students will point to various goals, such as studying for a test, but I ask about having sufficient attention simply to witness, or to be present to, life as it unfolds. What gets in the way of being present? For the yogi, we could say it is a complex of desire, judgment, control, and attachment: if I *judge* the present state of affairs to be 'bad,' I immediately *desire* to take *control* to make things better, and *attach* myself to the outcome. Alternatively, the true self is non-desirous, non-judgmental, non-controlling, and non-attached.

The journey toward the true self, then, is about a journey away from desire, judgment, control, and attachment. It is about detaching ourselves from all of these modalities of existing. But, in detaching ourselves in this way, we find ourselves not detached from reality but rather one with it, in the final limb of yoga, *samadhi* – an experience of the oneness of all, and one's continuity with all that is.

My focus when teaching *asana* is on differentiating the visible, objective body available to our senses and the invisible, experienced, subjective body available to the witnessing true self. By turning our attention from the objective body, which spurs in us so much desire, judgment, and control, to the subjective body, students experientially gain insight into what it would mean to identify with the witnessing true self.

Depending on your confidence and experience with yoga, there are many possibilities in teaching *asana*, from simply guiding your students to stand attentively in one place in *tadasana* (mountain pose) to leading them through a full yoga class, or even practicing *yogasana* with them throughout the entire semester. Because I'm not personally trained as a yoga instructor (and I suspect many of you are not either), I usually only engage them in a few poses and, alas, despite the title of this essay, I've never asked any of my students to touch their toes!

Mountain Pose (*Tadasana*)

In fact, to rule out the risk of injury, I usually stick to balancing poses, avoiding stretching altogether. I always begin with *tadasana*, just to get students accustomed to bringing awareness to their bodies. I ask them to close or lower their eyes and first of all just notice their alignment, without judging or trying to control it – just noting which side they are leaning toward, right or left, front or back.... Inevitably they'll begin adjusting their posture to how they imagine it's supposed to be (e.g., squaring and pulling back shoulders). We discuss how unnatural it feels simply to be non-judgmentally present, how quickly our judgments kick in, and explore whether it's possible to be free from judgment by attempting to be so directly.

Tree Pose (*Vrikshasana*)

Starting in mountain pose, the students lift one foot off the ground, at first placing the lifted heel on their opposite ankle, eventually working their foot up to their calves, and, if possible (a lot rides on what kind of pants they are wearing that day!), above their knees. I ask them to focus on a single, unmoving object to aid their balance. After they've settled in a bit, it's time for them to close their eyes. Almost immediately, and with a laugh, they fall out of the pose. Here they learn that the chaotic everyday mind is unable to offer the same degree of stability as the eyes. That is, they gained stability in the pose when their eyes were open by staring at an immobile object in the room. When they closed their eyes, they no longer had the luxury of that immobility. I ask them why they couldn't just find something similarly immobile in their minds, and they're quick to respond that nothing stays still in the mind. I add: well, that's where yoga comes in...

Next, we begin to discuss strategies for focusing the mind in the pose, particularly visualization techniques. I ask them to visualize internally (not by setting an objective image ahead of them) a stalk through the central axis of their bodies that extends above their heads and down below the ground, spreading out as branches above and roots below. This takes some time, but eventually, when I ask them to close their eyes, to their amazement, they almost invariably can maintain their balance.

General Remarks on Philosophy and *Asana*

Imagine, I ask my students, a marriage counselor trying to heal a relationship with only one partner, the other refusing to attend the appointments. Surely some work can be done, but in the end the other partner will need to show up. In the case of philosophy, the two partners are the mind and the body. Certainly much attention has been devoted to analyzing, but also to healing, their relationship. But, in the end, both partners will need to be present at the appointments. Yet, I fail to see how Western philosophy has really made an effort to even *invite* the body to the appointments, much less listen to what it has to say. What philosopher ever asked us to rise up out of our chairs, or so much as drawn our attention to the feeling of their book in our hands? But really, why would we ever have imagined we could explore the relationship between the mind and the body... without the body?

I dream of an entire philosophy class in which we invite our bodies to participate in each philosophical deliberation and investigation through-out the entire class. We could explore the relationship not only between the mind and the body but between any of philosophy's many conceptual oppositions (good and evil, universal and particular, one and many, yin and yang...) by exploring the oppositions that structure yoga poses (upper and lower, front and back, left and right, inhale and exhale, tension and release, upside down and right side up...). This is itself an ancient art: in some Hatha yoga traditions, for example, the front of the body is associated with the individual and the back with the universal. Yogis have long known that in forward bends we close in on ourselves and in backbends we open and expose ourselves, vulnerable, to the world. Backbends generate strong feelings of fear and anger, two very philosophically relevant emotions. What could we learn about our relationship to the world not by staring at it as it goes by before us but by sitting on our knees, reaching back and grabbing our feet, arching back into camel pose, and staring at the world upside down and behind us?

In learning to breathe through an emotion-releasing back-bending or hip-opening pose, what could we learn about witnessing and wisely responding to an emotion, rather than impulsively reacting to it? What might we learn about freedom? But philosophically reflecting on oppositions also involves questioning them and the hierarchies they so often imply. Can yoga guide us here? What if, stuck at a philosophical standstill, we positioned ourselves and our students upside-down, with our arms acting as our legs and our hands as our feet? When we turn our bodies 'on our heads,' might we turn our problems on their heads as well? What about downward-facing dog, when both our lower and upper bodies are 'on equal footing' and neither any longer have any priority or privilege? What could we learn about democracy in downward-facing dog? What about a political philosophy class that begins with a long exploration of down-dog? How would Hobbes' *Leviathan* have turned out if the body on which its highly hierarchical state was modeled was in down-dog?

Western Philosophy: 2500 years of *Pratyahara?*

There is undoubtedly a tendency and a temptation on the part of philosophy teachers who teach about yoga (or Eastern philosophy in general), and often more generally on the part of Westerners who approach yoga and Eastern philosophy, to malign Western philosophy – as dualistic, violent, hierarchical, and, ultimately oppressive – and to seek and find everywhere its contrary in Eastern philosophy – as holistic, peaceful, egalitarian, and just. Western philosophy becomes the problem in this take, and Eastern philosophy the solution. But I like to entertain a third possibility – beyond either embracing *or* vilifying Western philosophy's dualism – namely, that Western philosophy has been a very long and intensive exploration of the yogic practice of *pratyahara*, wherein the yogi indeed draws her attention away from her sensory, bodily experience and retreats into the interiority of her mind.

But, whereas in Western philosophy *pratyahara* is an end in itself – once one has left one's senses behind and entered the realm of the mind, one's journey is complete – in yoga, it is one limb of a much larger journey. Indeed, Western philosophers have often described the journey away from the body and toward the mind as a journey home, to one's true self, but, as we have seen, in the yogic tradition, the mind is definitively not one's true self, even if the retreat into it is a necessary moment in one's longer, and more circuitous, journey home. In this third possibility then, if there is an error in Western philosophy, it is not its having retreated into the mind and turned its attention from the body, but rather its having seen in that gesture the end of its work. From the perspective of yoga, it is, as *pratyahara*, only a step along the way.

Now, at the point at which I make this case – that Western philosophy was a 2500-year-long exploration of *pratyahara* – my students are already very familiar with the tendency of Western philosophers to prioritize the mind over the body. We will, for example, have read Plato's *Phaedo*, wherein Socrates drinks hemlock poisoning after having been sentenced to death by the Athenian jury for corrupting the youth of Athens. Far from horrified at the prospect of death, Socrates makes the case to his friends that 'he who has lived as true philosopher has reason to be of good cheer when he is about to die.'[1] In short, his argument is that death consists in the separation – indeed the *liberation* – of the mind from the body,[2] and the philosopher has been seeking that liberation his whole life, by always turning from the false testimony of his senses. He is 'entirely concerned with the soul and not with the body.'[3] 'He would like, as far as he can, to be quit of the body and turn to the soul.'[4] 'In matters of this sort philosophers, above all other men, may be observed in every sort of way to dissever the soul from the body.'[5] He asks: 'have sight and hearing any truth in them? Are they not, as the poets are always telling us, inaccurate witnesses?'[6] 'The philosopher dishonors the body; his soul runs away from the body and desires to be alone by herself....'[7] For Socrates, in death alone is the philosopher's dream of *pratyahara* truly possible.[8]

Now, Western philosophy has taken innumerable twists and turns since the time of its Greek origins, and it is likely unfair to say, as did Emerson, that 'Plato is philosophy and philosophy is Plato' or that all Western philosophers share this commitment to sense withdrawal. Indeed, in one generation, with Aristotle, Plato's student, much greater emphasis was be placed on empirical, sensory experience. Yet Aristotle's highest vision for humanity was still the mind's reflecting solely on itself. One gets the sense that Western philosophy never really shakes off the model of *pratyahara* entirely.

Indeed, almost two thousand years after Socrates' death, René Descartes argued so intensely against trusting one's senses that he refused – at least until his mind could reassure him – to accept that the physical universe, including his body, even existed. If *pratyahara* details the journey from the body to the mind, and Socrates sought that journey in philosophy and death, for Descartes, *pratyahara* took its practitioner so far from its point of origin (the bodily senses) that it questions whether that point of origin, and hence the journey, even existed in the first place! Next, just as Aristotle challenged Plato's commitment to *pratyahara*, the empiricists challenged Descartes. But, for the empiricists, the body functioned merely as a starting point for its proper journey to the mind. In the nineteenth century, German philosopher Friedrich Nietzsche depicted the entire tradition of Western philosophy as 'despisers of the body,' and in the twentieth ecological philosophers sought the root of Western civilization's problematic relationship to nature in its philosophers' problematic relationship to the body.

It is no wonder that so many of us trained in Western philosophical traditions turned away from it and sought other traditions. But, if we interpret

Western philosophy as specializing in *pratyahara*, we are left with another option. We could wonder what advantages the perspective 2500 years of *pratyahara* has made possible for us, and what *we can bring yoga* as we return to its fold. That is, as we rejoin the larger project of yoga of which *pratyahara* was meant to be a part, and no longer decontextualize *pratyahara* as an end in itself, we could wonder what such an intense and consistent practice will offer yoga's other limbs, just as we might anticipate returning to our *asana* practice after a long (in this case, *very* long!) meditation retreat, giddy to see what gifts the retreat would have brought that practice...

Where Now?

We are all familiar with the physical, psychological, and spiritual benefits of yoga. But have we explored what it has to offer philosophy? Perhaps where yoga meets philosophy we are on the precipice of a whole new horizon of philosophical investigation, an entirely new epistemological strategy and philosophical methodology. On the side of yoga, what awaits that tradition if its long-lost tribe of *pratyahara* specialists once again contextualizes itself within its fold? On the side of teaching, I have found no deeper, faster, or more enjoyable manner to bring students into the heart of philosophical speculation than through teaching them yoga. Indeed, my most creative, exciting, and passionate philosophical class discussions have come about through doing so. Well, I wish you the best of luck with your students, convincing your dean you're not crazy when she walks by your classroom, and, most of all, with recontextualizing the *pratyahara* you've been practicing all these years into the larger fold of the yogic journey toward the true self. I'll see (be?) you there (here?)!

NOTES

1 Plato, *The Dialogues of Plato*, trans. Benjamin Jowett (New York: Random House, 1937), 63e.
2 Ibid., 64c.
3 Ibid., 64e.
4 Ibid., 65a.
5 Ibid., 67d.
6 Ibid., 65b.
7 Ibid., 65c.
8 Ibid., 66e.

CHAPTER 7

MAN A MACHINE, MAN A YOGI

Why Yoga's Critics will Come Around

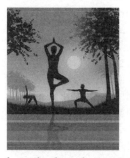 Depending on where you live, you may have had the following experience: You meet someone new and casually mention that you practice yoga, only to see the other person wince, smirk, gasp, or flee your company. At this point, it may have dawned on you that your admission has inadvertently betrayed you as (a) a New Age fad-chaser, (b) an immoral, unscientific body-worshipper, (c) a possible cult enthusiast, or (d) all of the above.[1] Whether you have had such an experience or not, it is apparent that yoga remains an exotic import in the West, not only because of its association with Eastern religion but also because it treats the mind and body as two perspectives on the same entity. The goal of this essay will be to explain why yoga is considered strange and controversial in this theoretical sense, and to argue that it should not be.

Classical Tradition

Speaking of yoga in the singular is misleading, as different schools emphasize different goals, interpretations, and practices. Some Western

Yoga – Philosophy for Everyone: Bending Mind and Body, First Edition.
Edited by Liz Stillwaggon Swan.
© 2012 John Wiley & Sons, Inc. Published 2012 by John Wiley & Sons, Inc.

schools offer only relaxation and health, whereas others promise enlightenment and access to the divine. When commentators and teachers try to speak generally about yoga, it is common to look back to the classical tradition and to *Raja*, or 'royal,' yoga, as many of the early principles, practices, and ethics announced then continue in various ways throughout contemporary yogic practices.

Written between 100 BCE and 500 CE, Patañjali's *Yoga Sutras* describes the Ashtanga, or eight-limbed practice, a program designed for those who seek *samadhi*, the binding of consciousness and integration of mind. This binding is not only the goal of yoga, Patañjali writes; it *is* yoga. The second sutra tells us 'the restraint of the modifications of the mind-stuff is Yoga.' For this reason, the word 'yoga' itself is often translated merely as 'union,' and the dualism of *Raja* emphasizes this union as the bringing together of *prakrti* (nature) and *purusha* (pure consciousness). *Prakrti* has connotations both of the contemporary English word 'nature' and of the more general notion of 'substance,' or fundamental stuff of the world. Consciousness, on the other hand, that feeling of 'I am' with all its manifold feelings, perceptions, memories, and stray thoughts, is enunciated only in multiples, finding only its true, authentic self in the union of yoga. The dualism of *Raja*, the dualism of yoga, is a unity of mind, but also of nature in the broadest sense of both the physical and of being. This insistence on the union of mind and nature is what makes yoga so controversial.

How does this union occur? Through practices that can be described, tentatively, as both mental and physical. These practices include meditation, the holding of physical postures, stretches, the uttering of the *mantra aum* ('om'), and a strict ethical code of duties and observances. Patañjali defines the nature of concentration as the 'binding of consciousness to a [unitary] place' and these practices are the means by which this binding occurs. Neither completely mental nor physical, these practices share the goal of a singular concentration in which *samadhi* can take place. This concentration emphasizes the non-distinction of mind and body. And, in the process of the binding of the conscious mind with *prakrti*, *samadhi* is attained, and the unity of things mental and physical is unveiled.

The *urdhva mukha svanasana*, or upward-facing dog – one of the more basic positions in yoga – is a good example of this. Your toes point back, your fingertips forward, your chin up and ahead, and your chest out. The arch of the spine opens the chest, spreading the collarbones, expanding the lungs, broadening the pectoral muscles. The position is

J. NEIL OTTE

entered into on an inhalation, and the oxygen, the stretch, and the position work together to energize one's body, freeing stresses that lodge themselves subconsciously in the muscles. Anyone who has held this position has also experienced its imposition on their feeling, conscious self, and is made aware of the 'mind of their body' and, often, the sudden invocation of memories and thoughts that can be unlocked by merely assuming the position.

Descartes: Minds as Captains, Bodies as Ships

Just as Hinduism had its reformist movements in the second and third centuries, in the sixteenth and seventeenth centuries in Europe, Christianity was experiencing a significant upset, culminating in a series of conflicts now known as the Wars of Religion. At issue was a theoretical and moral dispute that pitted Protestants against Catholics, and all of this in a time when political authority was rooted in a conception of divine authority. Amid this combusting powder keg, a few voices rose to argue for a radical enterprise: a scientific revolution. They argued not only that we needed to start doing the business of science but also that science had an authority to speak on certain issues (e.g., the movement of the planets and the nature of the self) that were hitherto exclusively overseen by the church. This new authority required a new vision of the world and of human nature, and nowhere was this new vision more persuasively argued than in the works of René Descartes.

What can be known with certainty? For Descartes, this was an urgent question, but one that still required reconciliation with the divine. In the coming scientific revolution, the question of authority had to be wrestled away from the church just enough so that important discoveries, for instance that the Earth revolves around the sun, could be debated without condemnation. But none of the proponents of this new movement wanted a complete break with church orthodoxy. To this end, Descartes' *Meditations on First Philosophy* argued for a worldview that would provide an uneasy truce in the war between scientific inquiry and religious authority, one that is still with us culturally in many ways today. Contrary to the teaching of Patañjali, this view held that there were two basic kinds of things in the world: minds and bodies. Bodies included all physical matter (e.g., human bodies, but also tables, chairs, stars, and pineapples) and were subject to the kind of physical laws that Isaac Newton would later formalize in his *Principia Mathematica*. Bodies were defined by their extension in space, and, as such, they could be infinitely combined, resorted, and divided. Minds, on the other hand, were known to us by the thoughts they experienced. These minds were described as extentionless, indestructible, and known only to their bearers (i.e., only you can truly know your own mind).

While this framework was controversial for years after Descartes' death, it was also clear that Descartes had stirred the intellectual imagination of Europe, giving it a new framework and a new set of problems. Perhaps the most pressing of these was what has come to be known as 'the mind–body problem.' Unlike Patañjali's *weak* dualism, wherein both mind and body are revealed in *samadhi* to be in unity, Descartes' dualism is *deep* in the sense that these two basically different things are ultimately irreconcilable. To understand the mind–body problem, then, it is perhaps best to recount what Descartes had achieved in his truce: Bodies could be the object of scientific inquiry, whereas minds were indestructible, completely free (as they are undetermined by physical laws), and could be handed over to the religious authorities, who were thought to know best about psychology, ethics, and that most mysterious of all things: the soul. On the face of it, then, it appeared Descartes had been quite successful in providing Westerners with a satisfactory division of labor, but such was not to be the case.

Descartes solicited responses to his *Meditations* from colleagues and soon cracks in the truce began to show. In her letters to Descartes, Elisabeth von der Pfalz, Princess of Bohemia, expressed skepticism about the separation of the mind and the body. If the mind and the body are completely distinct, she wondered, how is it that they can interact? How can an immaterial mind push a material body around, and how can a material body affect an immaterial mind? The interaction seemed unintelligible. Descartes struggled valiantly for an answer, but famously came up short.

Although Patañjali is deeply concerned with the mind and the body, the problem of their interaction would not have appeared to be a serious obstacle, but rather a failure of imagination. The mind and body in yoga are not distinct categories of being in a *deep* way, and the evidence for this is not in the form of a mathematical proof, but rather via an immediate, felt experience of oneness with all being. This difference in criteria of evidence stems from a disagreement about the nature of truth in yoga and in Western philosophy more generally. For Descartes, 'truth' is the

J. NEIL OTTE

word we give an idea due to its accurate reflection of some external state of affairs in the world, and, for Descartes, this accuracy can be described in words. For Patañjali, by contrast, truth is an authentic state of mind in oneness with nature in the broadest sense. As such, any use of language at all is immediately suspect, since language divides the world into subject and object, being and non-being, in any description. This fundamental disagreement about truth plagues East–West dialogue, and has certainly hindered the reception of yoga.

This is too bad, since it would appear that Patañjali's weak dualism is a more convincing answer to the mind–body problem than Descartes' desperate solution: that the pineal gland, which sits just above the cerebellum and is about the size of a pea, is the place where the mind interacts with the body. Descartes' reasoning for this conclusion seems to be two-fold. On the one hand, his autopsies of cadavers showed that the gland was singular and would have made a good place for communications received from the senses to converge (giving the mind a kind of 'mission control' from which to direct the body). On the other, it was possible that elements of the mind became very coarse, that the animal spirits became particularly fine, and that the mind is actually capable of directing the pineal gland to move these animal spirits in the proper direction.

This answer was hardly satisfactory, and, if two basic kinds of stuff appeared to be one too many, why not get rid of mind completely? One of my favorite thinkers who pursues this thesis is Julien Offray de La Mettrie, a physician and philosopher of the early half of the eighteenth century. La Mettrie saw Descartes as a closet materialist, or a secret proponent of the view that people are essentially physical, not ethereal spirits. His contention was not without reason. Descartes gives a mechanical analysis of the body, but La Mettrie took this analysis a step further and saw this mechanical description as accurately describing the workings of the mind as well. Descartes should have merely avoided the idea that the mind is distinct from the body. 'Is dualism still tenable?' asks La Mettrie. No!

What are human beings more like, then? La Mettrie provides two apt metaphors in his pseudonymous work, *Man a Machine, Man a Plant*, where he provides a completely physical description of the workings of the body, as well as the mind. Human beings are like plants, he tells us. Want to be healthy? Perhaps you require more sunshine, dryer air, and a less rainy climate. Or, perhaps your soul withers in the sunshine, and you require the foggy environs of mountains, lakesides, and streams. Man,

La Mettrie tells us, 'is an ambulatory plant who transplants himself. When the climate changes, naturally the plant sprouts or shrivels.' A careful rereading shows that La Mettrie's somewhat tongue-in-cheek descriptions are not too different from the sincere prescriptions of Patañjali, who specifies various ethical and daily practices for the purifying of the soul. Both describe goodness in terms of 'cleanliness' and 'purity,' and, while for Patañjali this state is divine whereas La Mettrie makes no such claims, they both agree to identify goodness with the health of the mind *and* body.

La Mettrie's amusing comparisons of human beings to machines and plants betray a real truth that is apparent to practitioners of yoga: our physical bodies have indelible impacts on our mental well-being. To Patañjali, as well as for contemporary yogis, this would be a truism, but to those for whom the mind was considered a separate entity, distinct from the body, this analysis was, if not completely novel, at least blasphemous. This was particularly the case when it came to sex, which La Mettrie thought both natural and necessary to health. Contrary to traditional sexual mores that held that the carnal desires of the body were to be resisted by a sufficiently strong spirit if the mind was to be kept pure, La Mettrie argues that avoiding sex can lead to disease. Discussing one particular female case, he writes, 'If her needs do not find prompt relief, the effects caused by uterine passion will not stop at mania, etc. No, this unfortunate woman will die of a disease for which there are physicians aplenty.'

This bawdy sentiment, combined with La Mettrie's crass materialism, caused scandal wherever it was received. Nonetheless, it was supported by the quickly maturing science of physiology. William Harvey, the English physician, in 1628 published his *De Motu Cordis* (*On the Motion of the Heart and Blood*), which accurately described the circulation of the blood throughout the body. Other innovations followed in La Mettrie's lifetime. In 1701, Giacomo Pylarini gave the first smallpox inoculations in Europe; in 1736, the French surgeon Claudius Aymand performed the first successful appendectomy; and, in 1747, Alberti von Haller's *Primae Lineae Physiologiae* – the first textbook on physiology – was published. These discoveries underscored the ability of modern medicine to achieve dramatic results by treating bodies as machines with interworking parts.

By the nineteenth century, Western medicine had adopted a strictly materialist orientation. No wonder, then, that yoga has received such a rocky reception.

Rejecting Descartes: Ships Passing in the Night

Douglas MacArthur famously said, 'Old soldiers never die; they just fade away.' In the history of philosophy, ideas are much like these old soldiers. Rarely do ideas die completely, though the ardor with which certain debates are pursued can flag as problems are solved, distinctions become reconciled, or the terms of the debate simply change.

In this sense, Descartes' distinction between the mind and the body is still very much alive in Western culture, particularly among the three Abrahamic religions of Judaism, Christianity, and Islam. Representatives from each religion have raised concerns about yoga's conflation of what they see as distinct parts of nature: minds and bodies. Recently, Southern Baptist Seminary President Albert Mohler condemned yoga along similar grounds, saying that he objects to 'the idea that the body is a vehicle for reaching consciousness with the divine.' In a blog post, he writes, 'There is nothing wrong with physical exercise, and yoga positions in themselves are not the main issue. But these positions are teaching postures with a spiritual purpose. Consider this – if you have to meditate intensely in order to achieve or to maintain a physical posture, it is no longer merely a physical posture.'[2] Mohler is concerned with the idea that yoga will somehow contaminate Christian minds, and that there is a hidden message within yoga to the effect that physical exercise can have a spiritual consequence. For Mohler, only a communion with a transcendent god is capable of providing human beings with spiritual sustenance, and the idea that the mind is positively affected by physical activity is a vain and blasphemous hope. The divinity of the union of consciousness and nature that Patañjali describes is, he thinks, incompatible with Christian doctrine.

The history of the mind–body problem in twentieth-century philosophy is long and complicated. Much of the early part of the century was concerned with rejecting the idea that we had anything like Descartes' mind at all. Behavioral psychologists attacked the notion of freedom, collecting empirical evidence to illustrate that behavior was a result of operant conditioning. The philosopher Ludwig Wittgenstein persuasively argued that language use was not, as had been thought, a decoding of private ideas, but rather a matter of public use, with the implication that meaning itself was not a magical thing belonging to mind alone but rather a continually disputed product of inter-subjective communication. These attacks on the 'realm of the mental' have persisted, but, rather than rehash the reasoning behind them here, I'll tell you a story.

When I was sixteen I visited the Veterans' Affairs Medical Center in Topeka, Kansas as part of a psychology fieldtrip. My teacher and a handful of students visited with the experts there, who talked to us about the kinds of treatment options available to returning soldiers, many of whom had issues with depression, post-traumatic stress disorder, anxiety, and other mental health issues. One of the psychologists allowed us to experience biofeedback. I was asked to lie back in a comfortable chair and to wear headphones while wearing an EKG helmet. The tape I heard was around twenty minutes long and contained a voice that slowly described the following scene: 'You are walking through a forest. You can feel the ground beneath your feet; hear the babbling of the creek and the chirping of birds. You see a cabin ahead of you.' All of this took perhaps ten minutes. Then the voiceover took an odd turn. 'You look up and see smoke rising from the chimney of the cabin, small wafts of smoke. You are that smoke.'

When I heard those words, I suddenly felt myself rise out of my own body and had the distinct feeling of turning and floating above myself. This feeling did not last long, but it was so incredibly strange that to this day I still remember it as though it had just happened. The question becomes then: What should I conclude? Was my mind rising up out of my body? Who is right here, Descartes or Patañjali?

These out-of-body experiences are not unique, nor are they supernatural. In chapter three of the *Yoga Sutras*, Patañjali describes this floating mind that can leave the body as a result of intense practice, but cautions that such experiences are merely a kind of distraction, and that the purpose of yoga is not to acquire such 'supernatural' powers but to relieve suffering in the world. Any discussion of out-of-body experiences is often cited as exhibit A of the quackery of yoga, but this inference ignores how well-documented out-of-body experiences are in contemporary Western science. Dr. James E. Whinnery, a chemistry professor at West Texas A&M University, has written about these phenomena in his work with fighter pilots, who frequently report finding themselves outside their bodies after being spun around in human centrifuges while testing the effects of g-forces on the body. Along with tunnel vision, an experience of bright light, vivid dreams, memory occurrences, and a feeling of floating, these subjects also reported vivid experiences of being outside their own bodies, often even looking back at themselves. Whinnery indicates that this alteration of the patient's proprioception (i.e., the sense of where in space one's body or body parts are) is a result of the physical strain on the brain, which during especially high g-forces is deprived of blood. Is it any wonder then that the intense ascetic practices of yogis can often result in similar reports?

In 2007, Henrik Ehrsson of the Institute of Neurology at University College London conducted an experiment designed to trick a subject's brain into producing a similar experience. The subject stands before a video camera whose image is projected into goggles worn by the subject. The effect is that one sees one's back a few feet ahead of one's own body. An experimenter then touches the back of the subject. These two sensations – sight and touch – are then relayed to the brain, creating the confusing mental sensation that one is being touched a few feet ahead of one's own body. This alteration of one's proprioception is dramatically displayed when the subject is asked to close her eyes and is then moved a few feet back before being asked to walk forward to their original position with their eyes open. Frequently, the subject walks back to the position where they felt themselves to be, not where they were actually standing.

What these experiences illustrate is that our own inner sense of our bodies, our proprioception, is subject to manipulation by neural stimulation of certain parts of the brain, whether through direct sensory manipulation or by bypassing the senses completely and engaging the neural paths directly. But all of this only illustrates that minds are firmly embodied. Perhaps Descartes' notion of mind still has an absolutely free will as it sits in the pineal gland, pulling the levers and gears that allow my body to move about. Well, here too, neurology has precluded this possibility, underscoring yoga's emphasis on our unity with physical nature.

This began early in the century with the work of Wilder Penfield, a Canadian neurosurgeon, who discovered that, when a mild electric current was applied to specific areas of a patient's brain, the patient would have willful dispositions, such as a desire for ice cream, or vivid memories: the smell of her grandmother's attic, for example, or a specific musical passage. This practice of electrically stimulating a patient's brain is now routinely performed by neurosurgeons as a way of locating the damaged parts of the brain without impairing the person's mental abilities, but it also underscores a significant point: our memories, like all mental events, are caused by brain activity. The argument for this is simple: If there isn't corresponding neural activity in the brain, there is no mental activity to speak of. All the empirical evidence bears this out, though how we are to interpret the evidence is up for grabs. On the one hand, it refutes *deep* dualism: Our mental selves are not independent of the physical mechanism of our brain. On the other hand, what are we then to say of the status of mental events such as memories, intentions, conscious states, and the like?

One popular response, following La Mettrie, is to deny that we have minds at all, and to say that the mind is, on close analysis, the brain, and that our thoughts depend solely on its physical substructure. This view has a popular analogue: the computer. Perhaps the mind is merely software and the brain is merely hardware. We don't think that software is a magical, otherworldly thing that can operate without hardware. While there are open arguments against this possibility, notice that computers have already overcome many of the hurdles Descartes thought impossible for machines: computers can respond intelligibly to commands (e.g., Google, find me that book on yoga! Done), solve complicated problems once believed solvable only by human beings (e.g., Gary Kasporov, checkmate), learn new behaviors not in their initial programming (e.g., welcome back to Amazon.com [your name]; those yoga mats you like are now on sale), and appear quite ready to overtake us even in more complicated tasks such as facial recognition. This notion of mind as an information processing system, consisting of mental states that cannot exist apart from their physical hardware, is a powerfully attractive image to contemporary thinkers, and frequently leads to skepticism or rejection of any theory (e.g., yoga) that is committed to the importance of the mental.

To recap, yoga has two primary lines of criticism: one, following Descartes, holds that there are two distinct realms of existence, a mental and a physical, which should not be conflated. This position, however, has fallen into disfavor with contemporary thinkers, as recent arguments and neurological evidence have conclusively shown that mental activity relies on brain activity. The second line of criticism, following La Mettrie, argues that we are really only physical beings, and that the mental is unimportant or, possibly even, nonexistent. This position has also faced significant criticism. Frequently, this criticism is phrased (all too simply) as a religious objection to a scientific conclusion, where the religious objection claims that science is merely a poor discipline for studying our moral, psychological, and *human* selves.

At this point, we might ask the question: What would an adequate worldview look like? This is where we can return to Patañjali with some profit. For practicing yogis, the term of art is not 'dependence' or 'independence,' but 'interdependence.' The mind and body are only distinct from the perspective of unbound conscious thought. When the mind is clear and is kept from seizing on individual objects, worries, fears, and fleeting thoughts, and is brought into focus with the body, one realizes the unity of our selves with nature. This view leaves room for both the postulates of science and the importance of mind, securing our psychological selves within the natural order of the cosmos without seeking to explain it away. Far from seeing our bodies as mere meaningless particles banging about in fields of force, philosophers are increasingly accepting a yogic view. If they succeed in convincing others, I argue, then, as the broader culture catches up, yoga should find a warmer acceptance.

Will yoga prevail against its critics? I believe yoga gives us an experienced sense that it must. This belief is not the result of naïve mysticism or an attraction to the novelty of a foreign practice. Rather, this belief is supported by the experience of yoga, as well as the yogic ethics of social engagement, where individual persons say to one another the traditional greeting, *namaste*, and, in doing so, acknowledge the shared divinity within the other.

NOTES

1 I know of one person of my own acquaintance who was once photographed for her local newspaper in a lotus position. A few days later her elderly parents received a cutout of the photo from one of their friends accompanied by a note that read: 'Dear Mr. and Mrs. X, I am sorry to inform you that your daughter has joined a cult....'
2 Albert Mohler, 'The subtle body – Should Christians practice yoga?' *AlbertMohler.com* (blog post, September 20, 2010, http://www.albertmohler.com/2010/09/20/the-subtle-body-should-christians-practice-yoga).

CHAPTER 8

YOGA FOR WOMEN?

The Problem of Beautiful Bodies

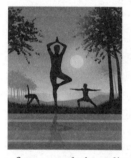

Yoga, as we commonly practice and understand it in the West, is a practice for the body. We are all familiar with yoga *asanas* (the poses of Hatha yoga); they are taught widely in gyms and yoga studios and increasingly have become part of popular culture: we see them practiced by celebrities and models and featured in advertising, in films, and on television. In addition, there are many yoga magazines, books, and DVDs, and hundreds of yoga websites displaying the yoga body. In this essay, I hope to draw attention to two concerns with respect to yoga's modern incarnation. First, how yoga has become a practice that is centered on the body and achieving body ideals, particularly with respect to women. And second, how yoga – a practice once considered an alternative to the materialistic confusion of modern life – has, in part, become consumed by the demands of consumer capitalism.

Yoga – Philosophy for Everyone: Bending Mind and Body, First Edition.
Edited by Liz Stillwaggon Swan.
© 2012 John Wiley & Sons, Inc. Published 2012 by John Wiley & Sons, Inc.

Yoga for Women?

Yoga is regarded in the West – much like aerobics and Pilates, which are also taught in group classes by an instructor – to be a primarily female pursuit. Girls, who it is assumed are reflective and quiet by nature, are suited to yoga, while boys presumably are more inclined to practice something more physical and 'masculine,' perhaps karate or kick-boxing. However, these gendered assumptions about who yoga is for are in fact a radical reversal of traditional yogic pedagogical practices. Hatha yoga, the physical practice of yoga with which we are most familiar in the West, focuses on the purification of the body in order to achieve purification of the mind. This practice, which originated in fifteenth-century India – although it has its roots in the eightfold or Ashtanga path of Raja yoga as described by Patañjali's *Yoga Sutras* (dating from between 100 BCE and 500 CE) – was traditionally taught from male teacher (or *guru*) to male student. Traditionally, *asanas* formed just one part of the yoga practice, which also included moral principles for living (*yama* and *niyama*), breathing techniques (*pranayama*), and different meditative practices and states. The purpose of the yoga practice was to gain control over the physical body so it could be used, through meditation, as a vehicle to achieve eventual spiritual enlightenment (*samadhi*); that is, union with the absolute or universal.

And so, male teachers passed on their yoga wisdom to their male students. This generally occurred between an individual teacher and an individual student. The male student worked diligently with his *guru*, often over many years, in an earnest spiritual quest to become a yogi. Women, meanwhile, were largely excluded from these lofty spiritual concerns. Seen as impure in Hindu and Brahman traditions, due to reproductive and sexual functions such as menstruation, pregnancy, and childbirth, women were considered unworthy for spiritual pursuits and relegated to the domestic sphere. Although there are a few stories and references to yoginis (female yogis) in the Vedas and later in Indian history, yoga was by and large a male practice and women were, for the most part, not invited or included.

However, it was a Western woman, Indra Devi, who is in part credited with spreading yoga, in particular the teachings of Krishnamacharya, to the West. Indra Devi was born Eugenie Peterson in Riga in 1899 and lived in Russia and Germany before moving to India in 1927, where she took her new name. Trained as an actress and a dancer, Devi starred in many Indian films. At a time when women were not normally accepted as yoga students, she persuaded Krishnamacharya – whose students included K. Pattabhi Jois and B. K. S. Iyengar – to be her teacher. Krishnamacharya encouraged Devi to become a teacher and she set up her first yoga center in Shanghai, where she lived with her diplomat husband. In 1947, she moved to California and founded a yoga school, becoming a yoga teacher to the stars. Over many years, she also traveled widely, teaching yoga wherever she went.

Devi's enormous popularity meant that, for the first time, yoga was introduced to the masses and, significant to the modern incarnation of yoga, to women. A glamorous socialite who was friends with many film stars, Devi opened her yoga studio in Hollywood, attracting people from all walks of life. Formerly a practice open only to men on a serious and rather ascetic spiritual path, yoga was now open to anyone who had the time and inclination to join a class. In fact, as Devi demonstrated with her great devotion to yoga and wisdom in its practice and teaching, yoga is an important and meaningful practice for women also.

Indeed, yoga as we know it today seems to be primarily a female practice, far from its masculine origins. Although there are many well-known male teachers and, of course, many male students of yoga, the majority of students and teachers in the West are women; in the United States, almost eighty percent of yoga practitioners are female. This is reflected in mainstream depictions of yoga practitioners: we see young women in yoga *asanas* in advertisements for cars, yogurt, health insurance, and a plethora of other products; we see beautiful women, the likes of Madonna and Scarlett Johansson, depicted as yoga teachers in Hollywood films; we see only women on *every* cover of *Yoga Journal* from 2003 to the present day.[1] Indeed, it is primarily images of women that feature in advertisements for yoga classes, yoga retreats, and yoga products.

However, this is not the only change to the face of yoga since it was taken up by Western practitioners. Taught in classes (rather than from master to disciple) and subsumed into the consumer capitalist logic of the modern Western era, yoga has become a practice for health and well-being, key values in late modernity, rather than a serious spiritual path to enlightenment. It seems that many women who have started practicing yoga have become fixated on transforming and sculpting the physical body through *asana* practice, worrying about burning calories, slimming down, and achieving visually impressive advanced poses. Hence, in an age where concern over the appearance of the body is paramount, the palpable physical benefits of a yoga *asana* practice have made it ever more popular and ever more marketable. As a result, the spiritual and practical aims of yoga have changed over the last century of practice as it has entered Western society. These changes are particularly significant for women and reflect broader social changes arising from the boom of consumer capitalism, concerns about the body as a 'project' and as 'capital,' the culture of celebrity, and the enormous growth of the fashion, health, and beauty industries.

The Yoga Body as 'Capital'

To say that yoga has proliferated in the West is an understatement. In contrast to perhaps comparable Eastern practices that involve mastery of a physical technique as a means to spiritual growth, such as tai chi, some martial arts, or chi gong, yoga enjoys an unprecedented popularity. In the United States alone, almost sixteen million people say they practice yoga, and there are millions more worldwide. Yoga is practiced everywhere: in studios, gyms, schools, hospitals, prisons, universities, and even in the White House. There are dozens of varieties, schools, and styles of yoga. But, as it has spread, yoga has changed. When it first arrived in the West, yoga was seen as a highly esoteric spiritual and cleansing practice; later it was regarded as a kind of preventative medicine to alleviate stress. The 'third wave' of yoga is the fitness wave, which is about losing weight and building strength, flexibility, and endurance. As such, yoga is nowadays regarded by many as merely a form of exercise that has the added benefit of calming the mind. Instrumental to this view of yoga has been the framework of consumer capitalism within which yoga has spread.

Consumer capitalism is not an incidental backdrop to changes in social practices and concerns, such as the transformation of yoga from a spiritual practice to a fitness practice, but rather often fuels, feeds, and informs these changes. To remain buoyant and viable, capitalist markets constantly colonize new territories, creating needs and desires that they duly serve. The body has become one of these new territories. The very lucrative fashion, health, and beauty industries have invested heavily in marketing the body as something that can be, and *should be*, changed, adorned, and worked on. Indeed, the logic of consumer capitalism infuses the body; it is increasingly seen as 'capital,'[2] and having the *right* body – slim, young, attractive, fit, fashionable – is increasingly seen as a means to success.

Hence, the body is not just something that I 'am,' but also something that I 'have'; it is seen as an 'investment.' Accruing 'body capital' plays an important role in most people's lives. Body capital includes 'assets' such as attractiveness, sexiness, style, and health, among others. Body capital increases one's 'market value' and one's chance for professional and personal success. The idea is, that the better I make my body – where 'better' is measured by norms usually proliferated by industries that stand to gain from people investing in their body-improvement products and services – the more wealth, success, happiness, and satisfaction I will find.

This sort of thinking is not arbitrary or employed by a superficial few. Empirical studies have shown that attractive people are perceived as possessing desirable characteristics and are treated more favorably and as more competent. It is widely believed that beautiful people earn more and have more successful lives: beautiful bodies, we see in almost every mainstream media, make *better* people who amass social and professional success. The bodily – and in particular a peculiar normalized hyper-attractiveness – seems to now serve as a sort of public signifier of one's social and moral worth. In fact, most people, if not all, believe that changing one's body can improve one's life.

These concerns around appearance and physical attractiveness are significantly, and, inarguably, more pronounced for women. Women have discerned that how they look affects how they are treated and thus their chances for success in various aspects of their lives. Indeed, in our image-saturated and digitally enhanced post-modern reality, physical attractiveness and beauty are paramount. We have learned to expect visual perfection and find any physical defect intolerable. As a result, the body has become a 'project' for women, something to be created, molded, and shaped. Over and over, we see that it is the smooth, toned, young, sexy, and glossy body that enjoys professional success and finds personal fulfillment. This perfect body is highly elusive and requires constant diligence, hard work, and enormous resources to be achieved. And, even then, it is most often an impossible ideal.

As a result, many women live in a constant state of frustration about their bodies. Under the veneer of freedom and success that modern Western women have achieved lie secret undercurrents of self-loathing, physical obsession, eating disorders, and a horror of aging. Constantly feeding these feelings of shame, inadequacy, and lack is the principle marketing strategy for the multi-billion-dollar beauty, health, and fashion industries. Cultivating profound anxieties about the body, these industries then present themselves as instruments able

LUNA DOLEZAL

to eliminate or alleviate the very shame and guilt they have themselves produced. Women are made to feel shame not only about their bodies (which, it is assumed, are not good enough the way they are) but also if they do not 'make an effort.' Consider the mantra of the cosmetics industrialist Helena Rubenstein: 'There are no ugly women, only lazy ones.' Internalizing this idea, many women spend a significant amount of time, energy, and material resources trying to achieve a socially pleasing body through various means: fashion, dieting, exercise, make-up, cosmetic surgery, beauty and skin products, and, in recent times, yoga.

Yoga as a Beauty Practice

Yoga, as it has come to be regarded as a fitness practice, has become just another product to be consumed in order to augment one's body capital. Indeed, as a form of exercise, yoga is highly effective. With regular practice, yoga practitioners find that the body becomes strong and flexible. Increasingly, as yoga has become a multi-billion-dollar, global industry, dozens of schools and styles of yoga compete for students, and dozens of companies trading yoga products compete for customers. As a result, selling the promise of the yoga body – slim, strong, flexible, young, poised, attractive, wholesome, hip – particularly to women, has become central to the modern incarnation of yoga.

One does not have to look far to see evidence of this change. *Yoga Journal*, which describes itself as the most widely read yoga magazine in the world, has started to compete with other women's glossy fashion and fitness magazines. In recent years, *Yoga Journal*'s cover invariably has displayed a poised and attractive yoga body adorned in fashionable yoga clothes and often positioned in a visually impressive advanced pose. (Interestingly, out of eighty-two such covers since 1999, seventy-five display women.) Through these sorts of images, which feature heavily inside the magazine's features and related advertisements, practicing yoga is implicitly related to attractiveness, affluence, and success. The message seems to be much the same as other women's glossies such as *Cosmopolitan*, *Elle*, or *Vogue*: If one can access and *buy* the right products – yoga clothes, classes, mats, retreats, DVDs, books, CDs, props, and so on – then one will augment one's body capital and, ultimately, success in all other aspects of life will follow.

Material success is an important theme of *Yoga Journal*, which often features articles on successful yoga entrepreneurs and, in addition, celebrities who have turned to yoga. In turn, yoga teachers, who achieve celebrity body ideals and popularity, enter the realm of celebrity themselves. Using elite film stars and models, who have seemingly ageless and improbably beautiful bodies, to represent yoga has been common practice since Devi used the actress and beauty icon Gloria Swanson to promote her yoga book *Forever Young, Forever Healthy* in 1953. For example, when *Time* magazine ran 'The Power of Yoga' as its cover story in 2001, it featured supermodel Christy Turlington – in the highly advanced posed *kukkutasana* – as the face of yoga. The enormous growth of the yoga industry in the West is perhaps due in part to attractive celebrities practicing yoga regularly and promoting it in interviews and lifestyle features. As a result, it seems that celebrity, yoga, and the beautiful body are a powerful, and increasingly popular, marketing trio.

Consequently, we find celebrities – a portion of society that notoriously, and publically, struggles with beauty and body ideals – becoming yoga teachers and yoga icons. It seems that, instead of forming an alternative to limiting and self-destructive body standards, yoga is subsumed into the same normalizing logic of other beauty practices. Indeed, a very recent trend in yoga advertising demonstrates how the yoga industry has begun employing the usual marketing strategies of the beauty, fashion, and fitness industries, cultivating feelings of shame and self-consciousness in women in order to boost sales. Lulu Lemon, a highly successful yoga clothing franchise, recently ran an advertisement that featured a woman in camel pose (*ustrasana*) with the caption 'Say No to Camel Toe,' a pun intended to provoke self-consciousness about the presentation of one's crotch area. Presumably, buying the (very expensive) yoga pants featured in the advertisement will alleviate these feelings of self-consciousness and allow one to get on with one's yoga practice with dignity and style.

In another recent advertising campaign, Toesox, a company that sells non-slip yoga socks, featured a series of black and white nude images of the yoga teacher Kathryn Budig. The images are very sexualized, presenting Budig's mostly naked body in a series of advanced poses. Using naked or half-naked women to advertise cosmetic, fashion, and fitness products is common practice, where normalized, and often sexualized, female forms are displayed in order to provoke feelings of inadequacy in women, ultimately boosting sales. However, this strategy is something new – and surprising – in the yoga world.

I do not mean to suggest that celebrity practitioners do not have enriching, meaningful, and spiritual yoga practices of their own. Nor to suggest that *Yoga Journal*'s editors have any conscious malicious intent toward their female readership. Nor do I hope to suggest that buying and using yoga products is in any way compromising to one's yoga practice. Indeed, as I know from my own experience, these products can often enhance or improve one's practice. Rather, I hope to draw attention to how yoga – a practice once considered an alternative to the materialistic confusion of modern life – has, in part, become consumed by market demands. Doing 'good' yoga has come to be equated with accruing body capital. It has come to mean proving one's physical adeptness through the mastery of advanced poses with the aim of sculpting a beautiful and youthful body. It has come to mean adorning this body with the *right* yoga clothes and accessories, displaying it on the *right* yoga mat, in the *right* studios and with the *right* teachers. But, can having strong abs, flexible hamstrings, and a fashionably attired yoga physique really help us cultivate an inner peacefulness that can help us live our lives with compassion, skill, and philosophical mindfulness?

Conclusion: Yoga for Every*body*

I hope to have suggested that there is something lost in the practice of yoga when it becomes merely an exercise system to promote a normalized body ideal. Yoga is a practice to end suffering, not by temporarily shaping the body to conform to pleasing normative body standards (which opens up the self for future suffering when the body inevitably ages and changes) but by delving into new experiences that cultivate equanimity, compassion, and an inner strength to face the inevitable vicissitudes of life.

Although Hatha yoga is a physical practice with palpable benefits in terms of flexibility, strength, muscle tone, coordination, and balance, it differs significantly from other forms of exercise taught in a comparable instructor-group setting, such as aerobics or Pilates. Yoga is not merely a physical endeavor with the aim of improving the body, but a multi-layered spiritual pursuit that includes moral codes and an earnest quest for spiritual fulfillment and eventual enlightenment. As such, the aim of a yoga practice is not to shape the external body through weight loss or muscle gain but rather to forge and deepen the connection between the body and mind through certain physical practices. The yoga practitioner, through his or her own yogic labors, builds body awareness through the practice of poses and breathing techniques. This mastery over the body comes from an *inner* awareness that culminates in a meditative practice. The yoga *asana* practice is merely a small portion of the traditional eight-limb yoga path described by Patañjali.

Indeed, it is thought by many that *asana* practice was developed solely to prepare the body for meditation: the poses open the hips and lengthen the hamstrings to facilitate a cross-legged seat; they strengthen the back and open the shoulders in order to maintain the spine upright. The breathing practices, cleansing techniques, seals, and locks balance the body energetically. With this balance comes a deep sense of well-being. It is perhaps for this reason that yoga initially enjoyed much popularity in modern times. As people feel increasingly alienated from their bodies, yoga offers Westerners a means to develop a relationship and inner connection with themselves outside of the turmoil and confusion of modern life. With this connection comes a sense of comfort, well-being, and lasting happiness.

Helping to shift emotions, traumas, and behavioral patterns that are lodged in the physical body, yoga also has profound therapeutic benefits, both individually and collectively. Indeed, many yoga teachers are using yoga in community and humanitarian work as a tool for healing and transformation. For example, Project Air in Rwanda uses the practice of Ashtanga yoga to help HIV-positive women and girls who experienced sexual violence during the genocide of 1994. Other community yoga projects offer yoga to the homeless, to prisoners, to addicts, and to disadvantaged youths, among others. In helping to overcome limiting and negative ways of viewing the self and the body, yoga has profound transformative potential.

As such, yoga can be a practice that can help women find an alternative to the normalizing body pressures that infuse modern life. Instead of encouraging women to strive for impossible body ideals and perhaps turn to other body-shaping activities, such as dieting or cosmetic surgery, a yoga practice can cultivate acceptance and understanding with respect to the body. In yoga, the body is not seen as something to be trans-formed or shaped, but rather a laboratory through which one can gain a philosophical and spiritual understanding of the self. The practice of the yoga *asanas* provides an alternative and compassionate vocabulary with which one can regard the body and the self; this is a vocabulary beyond comparisons and criticisms. The body's uniqueness is not compared to some ideal; there is no such thing as too fat, too short, too tall in yoga. Beyond certain alignment principles in the poses, the body's appearance, in an aesthetic sense, is irrelevant. In fact, there is no attractive or ideal body; the poses act as templates, but there is no end goal, nor any external comparisons to be made. Unlike other physical practices and sports, yoga is not about comparisons and competition: every*body* can practice yoga. And, through this practice, transformation and healing can take place.

Hence, there is something truly amiss when yoga magazines, DVDs, teachers, and books employ the usual marketing strategies of the beauty, fashion, and fitness industries. Suggesting, as the advertisements for various yoga products do, that achieving 'balance,' 'beauty,' 'power,' 'wonder,' 'grace,' 'poise,' and 'strength' will come from buying and using yoga products worn and displayed by attractive, often sexualized, young women whose bodies conform to normalized body ideals can only feed feelings of inadequacy, shame, and frustration in women who are already perhaps struggling with these cultural pressures. The practice of yoga should, instead, alleviate these concerns regarding the body and invoke a greater compassion and understanding of the body as it is now, not as it might become. Fitness and increased body capital may accompany a spiritual journey in yoga, but they are by no means end goals to be pursued. Instead, a yoga practice can, and *should*, reach beyond the instant gratifications or fleeting pleasures of consumer capitalism, and bring a deep joy and lifelong embodied satisfaction.

NOTES

1 Since the time of writing, Los Angeles yoga teacher Matt Pesendian has appeared on the cover of the March 2011 issue of *Yoga Journal*. It was the first time in eight years that a man had been featured on the cover.
2 'Capital' is a term usually associated with exchange within the economic and financial sphere. However, the term has been employed symbolically and in a wider context to describe a system where various assets are traded or transformed within social networks of exchange and value. Whereas economic capital – for example, property, currency, or material assets – is immediately convertible into a monetary form, non-economic forms of capital, such as 'social capital' – which includes 'assets' such as education, skills, or class – operate on a system of cultural exchanges that are not easily reduced to a strict system of valuation.

CHAPTER 9

THE FEELING OF BEAUTY
A Yoga Project

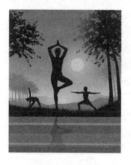

Experiment

On a crisp November morning, before participants arrive for the first day of shooting for the Real Beauty Yoga Project, I stand gazing at the items I've set out: two dozen red, coral, and yellow roses; one bunch of maroon gerbera daisies; a multitude of scarves and wraps; two pieces of reflective gold poster board to use as an outdoor lighting system; and a resin statue of green Tara – a Hindu deity revered as an eradicator of fear and a protector of women. Taking note of the objects spread like a color wheel across my leafy, overgrown backyard, an ocean of uncertainty swims through my belly, accompanied by the thought that I have placed myself, yet again, at the mercy of experiment. Following my enthusiasm with abandon, I've run smack into the moment where I must now discover what exactly I mean when I claim that today we will locate, express, and document the real living beauty of participating yoginis.

As my eyes land on the pointy black tip of Tara's crown – the same tip I gashed my forehead on earlier in the morning when I stumbled while carrying Tara and a host of items to the yard – I attempt to define real beauty. Immediately, I qualify in my mind what real beauty is not. I recall the shocking day of objectification and division inside a yoga studio that inspired me to begin a project devoted to documenting an expansive view of beauty within the world of yoga. My meandering thoughts are interrupted; the cold, wet grass touching my toes through my plastic yellow flip-flops makes me flinch. Looking down, I notice a single hydrangea flowerhead budding in the small garden bed by our garage where, last year, we failed to grow strawberries. The hydrangea is striking; it stands upright in a barren plot of dirt. Words cannot encapsulate my experience as I regard the sky blue petals in the morning air. Beauty that arises within an experience of immediate noticing is one way, perhaps, to name what I hope to document.

Cleo is the first to arrive. She has a spare frame, and penetrating black eyes. We sit on my flaking wood porch to meditate. After fifteen minutes, Cleo picks up a brass statue she's brought depicting Parvati, the Hindu goddess who represents Shakti, the feminine energy of the universe. This Parvati features ample round breasts and delicate waist beads around her belly. Looking closely at the statue's right hand, sculpted to drape softly over its bent knee, Cleo shares that Parvati is a totem of the beauty that inspires her. She adds that, when she acts from a mindset dominated by fear of lack, she perpetuates material lack, yet, when she assumes her life is already abundant, she tends to generate abundance. For Cleo, Parvati is the reminder of a life that is already rich. She twists her long legs into a seated posture two feet behind Parvati, and, like the statue, cocks her head to the side. I get my camera. We begin.

The second practitioner, Justine, lives in a straw bale home off the grid. For years, she has gathered her family's firewood and well water. She is the mother of a teenager, and enjoys her work as a yoga teacher and gardener. She keeps her dreadlocks long and does not shave or wax any body part. Sitting with her shoulders slightly curved, she shares that, even as she makes these choices from an empowered place, her confidence sometimes feels shaken by cultural dictates of beauty. I am surprised; Justine carries herself with an erect posture that conveys clarity and self-assurance. As if she can read my thoughts, she lengthens her spine and exclaims, 'Let's shoot my body hair! Natural is beautiful!'

Cleo, who has stayed to help, gets our cameras. Justine breathes steadily through a series of *asanas* while we use our reflective board to highlight the hair on her arms and legs. Snapping photos, laughing, and experimenting, all three of us begin to feel wide in this claiming we are doing – together – of beauty. One of the most stirring prints features

Justine smiling in *navasana*, or boat pose, with her feet facing the camera, leg hair in view, a maroon gerbera daisy sitting atop a bursting ponytail of dreadlocks.

Inspiration

My primary yoga teacher, Sofia Diaz, offers Hatha yoga as a sacred art. Practices with Sofia are devoted to the pervasive field of love shining within each being. Practicing yoga from this perspective has enacted a shift in how I feel about being alive. From day to day, I find my existence, and even my appearance, endearing. I'm often taken by others' unexpected beauty: my sixty-seven-year-old neighbor's flaxen hair flows in the wind when she waves and I see that she resembles the sun; my friend Natya crouches on spread feet to peer at dandelions popping up through sidewalk cracks and my mind pauses from a string of thoughts to notice her care.

Sofia has been fondly compared with Kali, the Hindu goddess of time, change, and destruction. In a clear and undaunted manner, she regularly confronts students by naming our 'punky resistance,' a term I understand to mean an avoidance of the strong sensations that arise when a student practices *asana* with enough intensity to amplify *prana*, or life force. Sofia does not rouse us to pump or push or sweat; she challenges us to feel. Her sequences often require students to hold *asanas* for durations that provoke remarkable feelings of vulnerability. After years of practice, I've been able to feel the stuck red pain of my own self-hatred, which peaked through years of severe anorexia as a teenager and young woman. Not easy. Yet, feeling this quality has finally given me the choice of letting it drop. Which has, in turn, informed my capacity to feel and express joy.

Sofia's *pranayama-asana* classes lead me to experience a sense of having nowhere to go and no way out. Her classes make use of vigorous body practice to help students intuit that the egoic mind cannot fashion a valid method to relieve itself of the limitation of life in a body. During moments when I have realized that I cannot avoid what I feel in one of Sofia's classes, I've experienced explosive sensations of terror, and simultaneous relief. Over time, this practice has broken through my resistance, leaving me open to the energy and light pulsing through my body. I have been lit with the sensation of being overwhelmingly in love.

My initial inspiration for the Real Beauty Yoga Project arose through a realization. Practicing yoga under Sofia's guidance had enacted a shift in my perception of beauty, from one that felt tethered to a cultural view to one that feels more observant and immediate. A single, disheartening day in a yoga teacher training course I completed from a different tradition provided a further impetus for the project. The studio hosting this program – at one time traditional and Ashtanga-based, but since transformed into a conglomerate of yogic offerings – needed a new studio brochure. I was absent when my fellow trainees agreed, as one student put it, to 'star' in a photo shoot.

This news left me with a dual emotional flavor of excitement and intimidation. Growing up in Los Angeles – a city engulfed in celebrity aspiration – made the moment familiar. Outwardly, I acted nonplussed. The troubling negotiation with power that accompanies fame feels as threatening to me as it does alluring. Feeling the fantasy of happiness-via-fame to be a trap for my dreamy mind, which routinely attaches itself to the narrow whims of my childhood, I tend to shy away from opportunities to be noticed. When my fellow students informed me of the photo shoot, our practice room became feverish with energy. Would turning us into models inspire the yogic qualities we were learning to live and teach?

When I arrived at the studio on modeling day, professional design consultants stood at the entrance holding monochrome shirts and pants made by the studio's clothing line. A woman I'd never met gazed at me and said, 'Small for the top?' She handed me a crisp white tank top. A fellow student, whom I'll call Elle, actually barked, 'You *can't* fit into a small.' My relationship with Elle was casual and friendly – attack was not part of our usual banter.

The consultant waved away her remark. 'Try the small,' she commanded. I squeezed into the tank top, and struggled to breathe. The shirt smashed my breasts into a flat pancake in front of my heart. 'Looks perfect,' the consultant said, shining me a pearly, albeit lackluster smile. 'What about your hair?' My thick multi-colored hair falls to my hips. With a half-smile, I strolled my smashed chest into our studio space and braided my hair down the back.

Inside, two fit photographers squatted before a group of huddled yogis and yoginis in training. 'Make like you're best friends!' the one with gelled hair shouted cheerfully. Yogis and yoginis tilted their heads and flashed white smiles. I unrolled my mat, fighting back tears. My close friend, a teacher assisting the course, came to sit at my mat. 'No big deal,' he comforted. 'It's just how people are.'

After he pointed out that I could approach this day with a light heart, as my heaviness was as much of a reaction as my classmates' reaction to potential fame, I too went over to hug myself into our flock. Still, I couldn't shake the thought that what we put our attention on, we become. When we put our attention on uniqueness, we see more of it. When the business of yoga choreographs situations to reveal an appearance of happiness (but not the real thing), a yoga class becomes a product for the 'good life.' When yoga-based media focuses on acrobatic poses performed by lithe bodies, people are reminded of physical imperfection and athletic inability; yoga, then, becomes one more method for attaining external perfection.

During our *asana* practice, photographers moved about shooting group images and kneeling before well-aligned practitioners. Though they emphasized certain yoginis, this part of the day felt the least manipulated. Every person was included. The *asana* class was not shifted for our new status; our teachers were careful to instruct and adjust our bodies as on any other day.

After the morning break, a finely-coiffed, high-heeled woman clacked across our hardwood floor and studied us, now clustered for a teaching on *savasana* – a pose often conducted at the end of class to allow for relaxation. Minutes later, the design consultants strode in and tapped the shoulders of the five thinnest and most symmetrically featured students, who ranged in age from eighteen to twenty-eight. Our class age ranged from eighteen to forty-five.

For two hours, the chosen five did a series of *asanas* and huddling for the photographer while the rest of us learned to conduct our future students in the art of letting go. From one perspective, we were the lucky ones. Master Ashtanga teacher Richard Freeman once said in class that it was important to attempt *asanas* one has not mastered. In his characteristic tone of dry humor, he added that, if we'd already mastered such challenging poses, we might be put on the cover of a yoga magazine, which would create a host of problems we didn't need. We were lucky, then, not to have to spend time in our minds rooting out the challenge of appearing desired, a state that our media-fed culture aggressively equates with happiness, but that rarely causes it.

Although I took Richard's wisdom as a consolation, few people in our cheery room looked content. Group members gazed at the selected few with faces that looked pained and dim. Some of my fellow trainees were young enough to still be defining themselves in the world. These women in particular, I felt, watched the favored students with faces of defeat.

The word yoga is often translated as 'to yolk,' or to couple opposites. '*Ha-tha*' often translates as sun-moon. Hatha yoga has the potential to unify the sun-moon, or right-left, energetic spheres in our bodies. Once these opposing aspects of life force arise in union via practice, a flood of energy shoots up the spine and out through the top of the head. This experience is described in myriad ways, one of them being *samadhi*, or divine absorption. Taking Hatha yoga, then, as a gateway to union with the divine, what transpired on modeling day – a supposed yoga lesson, but an actual enactment of separation between practitioners – was the opposite. Modeling day forced us to pay attention to certain practitioners, which literally divided us.

From this day forward, these five innocent practitioners would remain the yogis and yoginis chosen to represent an image of the 'yoga' we were learning to teach, based not on how adept they were at physical practice, not on the wisdom they had realized, nor on a group choice to put them forward as the best individuals to represent us. These five practitioners were elected to represent the yoga we were learning to teach because they were thin, young, and evenly proportioned. Hard as it was for the rest of us, I can't help but consider the social weight they were also asked, without much choice, to bear.

At lunch, I walked six blocks to my white rental car – marked with hard maroon berries from a shedding tree – to eat. I didn't feel affronted at not having been chosen, perhaps because I didn't expect to be chosen. But the dim look on my young cohorts' faces struck me deeply. I sat there, in the balmy heat of a perfect California day, sobbing behind the steering wheel. After the break, our head teacher sat before us with a hung and bothered posture. He looked as surprised by how the corporate studio heads had conducted the day as some of us were. 'I hope we won't have to spend much time processing this,' he said. 'I can tell you that this will not happen again.'

History

Visualizing the long robes, large bellies, and untamed hair of popular Indian gurus who arrived in the United States to teach Westerners the principles of a yogic life in the 1960s and 1970s makes the current yoga-glam movement appear new – one more avenue for our hungry market. Yet the initial ties between Hatha yoga in the West and a manufactured, slender appearance emerged before these gurus' arrival. The relationship between yoga and a thin body also has roots outside the West – as far back, in fact, as yoga's inception as an ascetic tradition.

In 1919, Pierre Bernard and his counterpart, Blanche DeVries, opened a yoga studio in Manhattan, and later a retreat center in upstate New York, where the teachers instructing *asana* classes were disproportionately thin and attractive.[1] Meditative Raja yoga was also afoot in the United States via teachers such as Swami Vivekananda. It was Hatha yoga, however, that drew a larger audience. In 1937, Pierre's half-nephew, Theos Bernard, hit the national newspaper and radio scene with an extraordinary capacity to contort his body and an appearance that recalls a bulk-less Arnold Schwarzenegger. A decade later, Indra Devi, the tiny, Latvian student of Sri T. Krishnamacharya, followed her guru's directive to teach and established a small Hatha yoga studio in Hollywood.[2] There is no evidence that Devi advertised Hatha yoga's purpose as weight loss or beauty enhancement; these benefits, however, were soon impressed upon an image-conscious Los Angeles public. Devi's clients included several celebrities.

Swami Prabhavanda – a Vedenta Swami who held a strong, moderately sized Los Angeles audience in the 1930s and 1940s – denounced Hatha yogis as 'the Olympic athletes of spiritual attainment.'[3] Interestingly, Georg Feuerstein uses the word 'adamantine' – which translates to unbreakable – to describe what even early Hatha yogis were attempting to do with their bodies. According to Feuerstein, Hatha yogis set out to 'bake the body'[4] of physical limitation; not to live into their nineties, nor to secure an exalted appearance, but to 'withstand the onslaught of transcendental realization.'[5] The goal of early Hatha yogis, then, was to clean the body of impurities so it could function as a viable ground for enlightenment. Taken from a Judeo-Christian perspective, which berates the body of its savage needs from atop the mind's moral tower, this goal is ripe for exploitation. A 'baked' body that is pure, cleaned out, and chastened replicates residual Puritan beauty ideals all too well. When I was seventeen, I bought a copper pendant carved with an image of the skeleton Buddha (who I thought was a skeletal monk) and wore my rust-colored totem around my neck for four years. To me, this ribbed, half-robed monk, who displayed unrivaled mastery over the insistent demands of a fleshy body, was the absolute image of my hunger for, and feeling of, beauty.

Though the ascetic yogis of India, who carry a long and respected renunciant tradition, are not out to thin or tone their bodies for appearance's sake, their emaciated state portrays a capacity for mastery over a ruffian mass of fat, blood, muscle, and marrow that a Judeo-Christian

NICOLE DUNAS

view prefers we rise above. When consumer media bolsters this preference with a barrage of lean bodies, it may feel natural to see the ascetic yogi as powerful, sinless, beautiful. His mastery *is* jaw dropping. Self-mortification *is* amazing. Yet the worldview that motivated yogis in India to surrender bodily needs to the divine in the name of liberation was not linked to an aesthetic corporeal ideal.

Hatha yogis and yoginis walk a fine line. Feuerstein calls it a razor's edge. The aim of Hatha yoga is an en-lighten-ment of the body; yet, if today's explosion of power yoga studios is any clue, Westerners are more likely to practice Hatha yoga to achieve a bodily state of perfection. To a certain degree, our motives may seem innocuous. Hatha yoga is diverse enough to answer a variety of needs, including healing the body of physical or psychosomatic injury. But, when physical accomplishment alone becomes our goal, negative consequences will inevitably parallel achievement.

After I had been teaching daily for several months, Sofia mentioned that my poses were looking too 'perfect.' She reminded me that it is not what I do, but how I do it. Though certain physical postures I practice may appear refined to an untrained eye, they are far from mastered. My breathing is too inconsistent. I experience an inkling of the muscular awareness necessary to call the postures I practice complete. Practicing and teaching in a self-directed way, I'd begun focusing on my external physicality at the expense of breath, intention, and surrender. Three months after Sofia mentioned this, I ripped a hamstring attachment, which had frayed after years of vinyasa practice. Without continual surrender to what is greater, and to the gaze of a competent teacher, *asana* practice can easily degrade into a technique for polishing the ego. When our minds notice achievement before breath or muscular sensation, injury is likely. I am often humbled. Though I desire to be free of social standards of achievement and beauty, and though I experience moments of freedom, I still often act to perfect the limitations I perceive in the flesh.

Inside the Beauty Question

Can beauty be called objective, as Immanuel Kant maintained, or is it in the eye of the beholder? The current media marketplace appears to side with Kant, with a twist that posits physical human beauty as fat-less and digitally remastered. Feminist Susan Bordo writes of a 1525-dollar bill published in *Harper's*, reflecting the cost of airbrushing Michelle Pfeifer's face.[6] No amount of human effort, then, can meet our social bar of perfection. The joy often portrayed on bony models' digitally remastered faces sends a message that, if we keep sweating on our hamster wheels and spending generously on products, we might realize an impossible ideal.

The mind–body dualistic split so common to Western thought (i.e., that the mind and body are separate entities, with the mind being active, awake, and masculine and the body being passive, feminine, and undermined by its own appetites) is so ingrained that I'm certain the orchestrators of modeling day failed to consider it. The fact that we were made the passive, feminine body by being given no directive part in how we would be photographed, nor in how the photographs would be used to generate a product for the studio's monetary gain, was lost in the promise of yoga fame.

In the West, beauty is often discussed without regard for the constructed framework it sits within. We remark that Angelina Jolie is beautiful, while Kathy Bates is a talented actress. Even those who resist these distinctions understand the nuance of this remark. But do we consider the throng of images that have gone into making such remarks comprehensible? Do we think about the superior and critical position we're put in when we react to an image that cannot react back? We fail to notice the inherent illusion that we're alone in our perception when we savor, contemplate, or reject a paper or electronic image.

In *The Spell of the Sensuous*, David Abram writes about the natural landscape as a lively, animate ecosystem that perceives us as we perceive it. Written and spoken language in the developed world, he maintains, function to deny reciprocity with nature whereas language in oral indigenous cultures depends on sensory participation with the natural world.[7] When I hear a rainstorm beat like pellets on a corrugated iron roof, the sound resonates with such energy I can't imagine stripping the experience down to my subjective awareness. I agree with Abram, who maintains that 'whatever we perceive is necessarily entwined with our own subjectivity, already blended with the dynamism of life and sentience.'[8] I began reading Abram's work after spending seven months teaching yoga in Bali. When Abram, who also spent time in Bali, returned to the United States, his highly developed sensual capacity went numb. When I returned, my sensitivity to nature also diminished as the power of my associations took hold of my thoughts.

NICOLE DUNAS

Abram writes:

> I returned to North America excited by the new sensibilities that had
> stirred in me – my new found awareness ... of the great potency of the land,
> and particularly of the keen intelligence of other animals, whose lives and
> cultures interpentrate our own. I startled neighbors by chattering with
> squirrels, who swiftly climbed down the trunks of their trees and across
> lawns to banter with me ... Yet, very gradually, I began to lose my sense of
> the animals' own awareness ... I found myself now observing the [squirrels]
> from outside [their] world ... my attention was quickly deflected by
> internal, verbal deliberations of one sort or another ... by a conversation
> I now seemed to carry on entirely within myself.[9]

As Abram reimmersed himself in our literate culture's worldview, which
largely holds the animate world as a mechanical set of systems we can
abstract and control, he became unable to encounter the animate world
on its own terms. Similarly, when we objectify beauty into something
we merely gaze at, we lose our capacity to participate in beauty as
a mysterious unfolding. The more we objectify beauty, the more we
perceive it as separate from ourselves. Bordo reports that cosmetic
surgeons are all too familiar with the pattern of an isolated gaze: the more
cosmetic surgery women have, the more imperfection they see.[10] What
we put our attention on, we become. This aspect of our minds, when
preyed on, supports consumer capitalism.

I feel beauty most clearly through experiences that require conscious
participation between my perceptive awareness and the natural world.
I experience a glistening drop of dew on a purple-tinged Sycamore leaf as a
more visceral enactment of beauty than a magazine image, which represents
an experience unrelated to the one I am having when I look at the image.
The experience of yoga in my body – the enlivening quality of light moving
along my spine, or the raw feeling of an open heart in a fish pose, resonates
as a greater utterance of beauty than a commodified standard.

In *Yoga, Science of the Soul*, Osho's translation of the first yoga sutra
reads: 'Now, the discipline of yoga.'[11] Yoga happens in the present. Our
experience of yoga isn't fashioned from what we read, nor created by an
ideal image, as suggested by the teacher-training brochure where my own
smiling face appears. Similarly, a fair consideration of beauty honors
bringing oneself *now*, to the question of beauty. What arises in our
awareness that gives us cause to celebrate? What arises that strikes us as
beautiful?

A participatory experience of beauty is in greater alignment with Hatha yoga than an experience of beauty formed from a magazine image, perhaps for obvious reasons. The lived practice of Hatha yoga occurs in the present. A commodified view, feeding on greed, opposes the *Yoga Sutras*, which name greed as an *avidya*, or an aspect of ignorance yogis practice to overcome. A magazine ad is designed to fill our minds with notions of a product and how to acquire it – whether it's a high-quality yoga mat or an appearance of peace. This mind-patterning activity opposes yogic action designed to interrupt our habitual mind-flow, either to experience the body as light or to perceive reality as it exists.

Hatha yoga's tantric nature – namely, the assertion that liberation occurs via the body – contradicts the wound, I will say, of a dualistic Western view that faults the body as a hindrance to transcendence. I believe that this notion informs Hatha yoga's strong presence in the West. The celebration of the transcendent possibility *within* the body, so integral to Tantra and Hatha yoga, encourages yogis and yoginis to hold our bodies in kindness. We who have suffered a culturally induced criminalization of the body are hungry to experience our body as friend.

The Real Beauty Yoga Project is one attempt to explore a language of beauty that embraces, rather than divides, by asking individuals to place their expression of beauty at the forefront of an image-making process. At dusk, on that crisp November day, Cleo pointed her lens at me. Though I hadn't planned to be a subject, I tucked flowers between my fingers, stood by Tara, and moved into practice. Three-part breath. My cheeks flushed as I heard the camera click. Downward dog. My muscles sung with relief. Triangle pose. Headstand. Cleo scooped up daisies and tucked one between each of my toes. The stems were slippery. I didn't know if I could hold them. I had to trust that I could. And that Cleo's imagination was leading us down a road of beauty.

NOTES

1 Stefanie Syman, *The Subtle Body, The Story of Yoga in America* (New York: Farrar, Strous and Giroux, 2010), pp. 80, 99, 100.
2 Syman, *The Subtle* Body, p. 180.
3 Syman, *The Subtle* Body, p. 167.
4 Georg Feuerstein, *The Yoga Tradition, Its History, Literature, Philosophy and Practice* (Prescott, AZ: Hohm Press, 1998), p. 383.
5 Feuerstein, *The Yoga Tradition*, p. 29.

NICOLE DUNAS

6 Susan Bordo, *Unbearable Weight, Feminism, Western Culture and the Body* (Berkeley, CA: University of California Press, 2003), p. xviii.
7 David Abram, *The Spell of the Sensuous* (New York: Vintage Books, 1998).
8 Abram, *The Spell of the Sensuous*, p. 34.
9 Abram, *The Spell of the Sensuous*, p. 25.
10 Bordo, *Unbearable Weight*, p. xvii.
11 Osho, *Yoga: The Science of the Soul* (New York: St. Martin's Press, 2002), p. 2.

CHAPTER 10

PICTURING YOGA

Yoga Journal and the Perfect Form

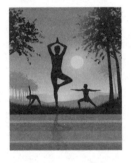

Introduction

Over the past fifteen years, yoga has taken the West by storm. Worldwide, as many as forty million people practice yoga and almost half of them are American. Some do it to relax, others for exercise and health, and some use it as a path to spiritual enlightenment. Once viewed as the strange behavior of contortionists, today yoga has become mainstream. Madonna recorded a song about her favorite form of yoga on her 1998 *Ray of Light* album; the Los Angeles Lakers take a couple of classes a week; Gwyneth Paltrow, Ricky Martin, and Meg Ryan are all big fans; and paparazzi perpetually snap photos of the famous coming and going from yoga classes. The fit and flexible teachers and students 'doing' yoga today are mostly women found in classes held at yoga studios, health clubs, YMCAs, and on college campuses.

In incarnations ranging from strict adherence to a prescribed series of physical poses to hybrid combinations of yoga, aerobics, and Pilates, the 4000-plus-year-old combination of philosophy and physical pursuit has a secure toehold in modern American culture. Growth in participation

Yoga – Philosophy for Everyone: Bending Mind and Body, First Edition.
Edited by Liz Stillwaggon Swan.
© 2012 John Wiley & Sons, Inc. Published 2012 by John Wiley & Sons, Inc.

has been rapid. Between 1990 and 1999, for example, the average frequency of participation in yoga increased from once or twice a week to about four or five times. Three million report attending a yoga class more often than twice a week. In the United Kingdom more than a half a million people are practicing yoga.

As with many things in the West, if there is an interest, there is a magazine to represent it, and yoga in the United States is no exception. *Yoga Journal* (*YJ*), established in 1975, grew alongside the interest in the United States in this physical and spiritual pursuit. Starting out as a small, ten-page magazine circulated to only 300 readers, *YJ* today enjoys a circulation of more than 350,000 and has an estimated pass-along readership (those who don't buy but otherwise come across the magazine) of one million. One might wonder, then, how *YJ* represents yoga on its covers. This is the subject of this chapter. If covers are windows to what is inside a magazine, what, in *YJ*'s case, are readers seeing? While voices of yoga's ancient traditions of practice (physical postures combined with mental discipline) still echo throughout some yoga studios today, they are much quieter in their post-colonial form and have been replaced in part by the West's emphasis on fitness, finance, and appearance.

By analyzing the magazine's cover images according to sex, race, pose, and appearance, this study explores how yoga is represented in the United States. Fifty-two covers of *YJ*, from between 2000 and 2008, were examined in order to answer the research question: How does *YJ* represent American yoga? Specifically, do the covers of yoga's primary publication reflect yoga's past (emphasis on equity, equanimity, equipoise, and equality) or yoga's present (models, marketing, and merchandise)? Featured on a 2001 cover of *Time* magazine, Western yoga's mind–body duality was demonstrated convincingly by supermodel Christy Turlington, whose limbs were entwined with the following text: 'Millions of Americans are discovering this ancient exercise. Here's the skinny on why it makes you feel so good.' Julia Roberts' response to questions in *InStyle* magazine about her involvement in yoga provides another clue: 'I don't want it to change my life,' Roberts said, 'just my butt.'[1]

This study is a response to the need for more magazine cover analysis and extends this area of research beyond some of the more typically examined covers such as *Cosmo*, *Life*, *Maxim*, and *Time*. Unlike truly secular publications such as *Cosmopolitan* or *Maxim* or *Sports Illustrated*, whose covers have been studied for their race and gender representations, *YJ* is anchored in a spiritual (while not religious) basis with content that speaks to its ancient origins. This is an important difference. While many studies have examined magazine covers in terms of sexual and gender stereotypes as indicators of editorial direction, few to none have explored the relationship between a cover image and philosophical continuity or integrity when the publication is about a philosophy and belief. Research on the ethics of digital manipulation of photography, such as on the cover of *National Geographic*, for example, comes the closest to exploring this ethical dilemma of reader-expected integrity and corporate need for sales. This approach to visual image research speaks to the unique place occupied by yoga as a physical pursuit nested in a philosophical system and situates the publication in a specific economic, cultural, and social context. Therefore, this study contributes to the literature on magazine covers and racial and sexual stereotypes. Do esoteric, ethically based titles have a special responsibility to their readers to present a less decorative and more multi-cultural cover?

Yoga, Magazines, and *Yoga Journal*

Yoga, as practiced in the West, is big business. Americans spend more than six billion dollars a year on classes, clothing, props, books, CDs, and practice mats. Besides its therapeutic, athletic, and spiritualistic boon, yoga offers something else valued in Western culture – the opportunity to make a profit and use sex to sell it. Representing a multi-billion-dollar market in yoga-related products, yoga practitioners are devoted to the practice as well as to consuming the related products. As described by a *Globe and Mail* (Toronto) reporter, a yoga class is a potentially profitable place for those in search of perfect bodies, perfect forms, and the inspiration for perfect bottom lines; that is, 'moolah yoga':

> And so it was that during the Battle of Conrad, in the Week of the Poisoned Dogfood, I took to my sanctuary, the cathedral of hotness known to the men and women in the City of Tightness as Downward Dog, to do yoga. And as I assumed the first *asana*, the pose of *voyeurata* – flat out on a green rubber mat, stretching the legs and peeping slyly at the lycra-ed beauties nearby – a corona of enlightenment inflated the room. And the vision was this: *Jesus, if I were in the yoga business, I could be making a fortune.*[2]

With its foundation in ancient texts that have modern pluralistic relevance, yoga appeals to modern interests in religious, philosophical, and spiritual syncretism but lacks the dogma of organized religions.

DEBRA MERSKIN

Ancient vows of asceticism and poverty aren't apt descriptors of today's practitioners. Those able to extend the time and effort necessary to fully explore the practice therefore tend to be educated and have the financial resources, time, and energy to look at spirituality in a comparative sense. What do yoga teachers and students look like? From the turn of the century until the early 1970s, the image was probably that of a bearded older man dressed in a simple white tunic or loincloth, seated in full lotus position or contorted into an exotic position, dispensing the secrets of the universe. Loyal devotees of the philosophical and spiritual practice were equally ascetic – limiting their diets, thoughts, and attachments to the here and now, and bending and twisting themselves into demanding poses designed to liberate their minds from the multitude of competing thoughts as well as strengthen and tire their bodies in order to sit calmly for meditation.

Today, seventy-three percent of yoga participants are women. Forty-one percent are aged between eighteen and thirty-four and forty-one percent are aged between thirty-five and fifty-four. Eighteen percent of practitioners are over age fifty-five. The yoga crowd in the United States is college educated, many with annual household incomes at or above 75,000 dollars and nearly a quarter with incomes that exceeded 100,000 dollars.[3] With all this money flowing and interest growing, it would make sense, in the United States, that there would be an associated publication, and yoga is no exception. The next section briefly describes American yoga's commercial and spiritual treatise, *Yoga Journal*.

Yoga Journal, founded in 1975 by the California Yoga Teachers Association, was the first magazine dedicated entirely to the practice of yoga and has the highest circulation among magazines devoted solely to yoga. Circulation built slowly and steadily and by 1990 had reached 55,000. By 1995, the figure was nearly 70,000. After a change in ownership, editors, and appearance in 2000, *YJ* was relaunched and today the magazine has a readership of more than one million as well as business interests in yoga retreats and conferences around the world. According to its editorial submission guidelines:

> *Yoga Journal* covers the practice and philosophy of yoga. In particular we welcome articles on the following themes:
>
> (1) Leaders, spokespersons, and visionaries in the yoga community;
> (2) The practice of Hatha yoga;

(3)   Applications of yoga to everyday life (e.g., relationships, social issues, livelihood);
(4)   Hatha yoga anatomy and kinesiology, and therapeutic yoga;
(5)   Nutrition and diet, cooking, and natural skin and body care.

The monthly magazine contains 'material that combines the essence of classical yoga with the latest understanding of modern science.' According to its website (www.yogajournal.com), *YJ* offers advice on poses; ideas about yogic philosophy; tips about diet and nutrition; reviews of yoga-related books, music, and DVDs; and extensive discussions of yoga styles and detailing of postures. It is dedicated to providing 'readers [with] insightful articles on yoga, filled with the most current scientific information available, while honoring the 5,000-year-old tradition on which it is based.'[4] The magazine is owned by California-based Active Interest Media, which also publishes *Backpacker, Southwest Art, Vegetarian Times, Yachts,* and other titles.

It is widely documented that bodies, particularly women's bodies, are used to sell products and services. Whether on or between the covers of magazines, the female form has been one of the most powerful sales tools used by publications and advertisers. The sexual objectification of women's bodies on the covers of magazines that target men such as *Maxim* and *Sports Illustrated* has been well-documented, as have the potential effects this form of representation has on the way men view women and women view themselves. The use of women's bodies as decorative objects on the covers of magazines whose editorial intent is intended to entertain and titillate, such as *Cosmopolitan, Maxim,* and sports-oriented publications such as the *Sports Illustrated* swimsuit issue, is not entirely unexpected nor necessarily out of line with the publications' editorial directions. From the magazine production side, whether the magazine is *Cosmopolitan, Maxim,* or *Prevention,* there is a consistent cover formula that relies on sexy women. In the same spirit, each month a different individual is presented on the *YJ* cover, demonstrating a featured pose. If eighty percent of newsstand sales are determined by what is on a magazine's cover, what is *YJ* selling?

Research Question

A magazine's cover is significant – it not only operates as an advertisement for the publication but also contributes to the visual landscape when seen in stores and at newsstands. Based on previous studies of magazine covers, the following research question motivated this study: does yoga's primary publication, *YJ*, reflect the practice's past or modern preoccupations with appearance?

Method

Two researchers independently analyzed 52 covers of *YJ* for the period 2001–2008. Cover images were obtained from the magazine's website under a link for ordering back issues. Two covers were obtained using Google's 'image' search engine. In conducting the research, I contacted *YJ* by email with questions about art direction and cover decisions, but my inquiries never received a response.

Both statistics and written descriptions are provided as part of this visual analysis. Coding categories were developed based on those originally described in Goffman's seminal work on gender and advertising. Coding categories for race/ethnicity and hair color (which can be suggestive of race/ethnicity) were added to the present study.[5] Cover models were coded according to the following variables: (1) sex of model(s), (2) hair color (blonde, brown, red, black, can't tell), (3) number of cover models, (4) race, and (5) portrayal (body view, pose, style and amount of clothing, sexual tone). Body view was coded as full (and three-quarter), head and torso, or face (head and shoulders). Pose was coded as standing, sitting, reclining, or face only. The amount of clothing was coded as nude, suggestive, demure, or partially clad. Sexual tone or sexiness was based on a combination of factors, such as whether or not the model(s) made eye contact and the effect of dress, pose, and expressions.

Results

All models on the 52 covers of *YJ* between 2000 and 2008 were white and only one issue had more than one model on the cover, for a total of 53 models. The single cover with more than one individual consisted of a photograph of a man and a woman. The man is seated in full-lotus and the woman is also in this pose, but on top of his shoulders. Two covers showed individual men (April 2001 and April 2003). Only one cover (December 2006) presented a celebrity teacher (Seane Corn).

In terms of body view, in ninety-six percent of the cover photographs, models' complete bodies were shown. Only two covers limited the image to the head and torso. According to magazine research, a 'life-sized human face looking directly at the viewer/reader' is critical for reader identification.[6] However, less than one third of the models looked directly at the implied viewer. Others were shown in profile or looking away. In terms of clothing, in most cases the body of the model was fully covered; thus, even if in leotards or other tight-fitting apparel, dress was coded as demure. Thirty-two percent of the cover models were coded as suggestively dressed on the basis of midriff- or cleavage-revealing bodywear.

Sexual tone or sexiness was based on a combination of factors such as whether or not the model(s) made eye contact along with the effect of dress, pose, and expressions. As mentioned above, the majority of models looked away from the implied viewer. The Gestalt of the cover image resulted in most covers being coded as not sexy (sixty-two percent). However, somewhat sexy or enticing covers were coded as 'yes.'

Implications and Conclusion

Magazine covers not only offer information about what's inside a particular issue but also provide significant cultural cues about the social, political, economic, and medical trends of a particular time – that is, context. To revisit the research question, 'How does YJ represent American yoga?,' this study shows the magazine to be consistent with other magazines that emphasize idealized white female beauty. The choice of yoga pose demonstrated by the cover model reveals something about the availability and openness of the person observed, but also reveals that she is posed as 'unaware' of the voyeuristic gaze of the reader. This code and convention of gender display presents the model as engaged in an activity and unaware of the viewer, who can gaze reassured of anonymity. This hierarchical gaze thus puts the model in a position of vulnerability. Yoga practitioner and scholar T. K. V. Desikachar noted that 'yoga is the practice of observing oneself without judgment' and is experienced 'inside, deep within our being.'[7] However internal the ideal process may be, scopophilic (deriving pleasure from looking) external evaluation is part of the set-up. In other words, based on the analysis of YJ's covers, it would seem that not only is achievement of spiritual enlightenment an elusive ideal but so is the attainment of the body

DEBRA MERSKIN

necessary to take one on that journey. The lack of racial diversity on the cover of *YJ* speaks to the idealization of yoga in the United States as a raced activity. Thus, white is reified as the default race. Cover models might wear a range of hair colors, but skin tone is the same, signifying a construction of beauty that values one type of woman more than others. In addition, while the 'repetitive cover formula' of *YJ* appeals to men because of the idealization of white women as a beauty norm and to women because of the familiarity of that 'sell,' this representation contributes to the perpetuation of yoga as a women-only activity.

The intent of this analysis was to decode the covers of *YJ* in order to destabilize the taken-for-granted nature of everyday media images, which sustain inequities that marginalize the interests and abilities of women and other minorities. Media texts are created to generate profits for the companies that produce them. Ideological themes such as those about ideal female beauty are encoded to create and appeal to niche audiences and encourage spending and consumption by these audiences. While audiences are able and always free to read media messages in multiple ways, there is always a mainstream presentation that is consistent with the priorities of dominant culture. Magazines are complex systems that use symbolism, and magazine covers are created in ways that contribute to an *idea* of a publication, one the reader can relate to. Through color, copy, and content, a design code contributes to the meaning of a cover image, a 'montage' effect, in which meaning is created by what is seen and what is culturally understood.

In order to survive, *YJ* must attract readers for its advertising. A consistent look, with expected colors and images and texts, builds the graphic identity of every publication. As a result, whatever ideology a magazine professes is invariably produced by, and a result of, its commercial context. Should publications such as *YJ* deliver more in this regard? Do readers expect more? Meanings are never neutral or only textual; they are socio-political. The decision of who models American yoga plays a powerful role in the communication of yoga's ideas, audiences, and benefits.

Communications theories and research show that what we see in the media at least contributes to, if not constructs, how we feel about ourselves, our bodies, our minds, and how we see those around us. Power is displayed and reified through beauty and can be used to manipulate. Admiration and emulation are often the result of these kinds of displays. Thus, the visual representation of mind–body integrative practice such as yoga, an activity that advocates for a strong, powerful, flexible body and a mind that is not preoccupied with unrealistic beauty standards, bodily comparisons, and exclusivity, carries with it responsibility – we both see and are seen.

René Descartes' seventeenth-century metaphysical divide between mind and body is inconsistent with the findings of modern neuroscience that demonstrate the intricate and intimate relationship between the two. Yoga's connection with improved health is well researched and it continues to prove itself as a powerful activity to help individuals dealing with health concerns ranging from attention deficit disorder to high blood pressure and body image issues. A disproportionate number of African Americans, for example, suffer from stress-related illnesses such as hypertension stemming from factors such as racism, poverty, and violent environments. Yet, participation in yoga by African Americans and other minority group members has lagged far behind that of whites. As one yoga instructor pointed out,

> Yoga changes lives. One of my goals as a teacher of yoga has been to bring yoga to the African American community. When I started teaching more than 20 years ago, all of my students were white. Certainly I wanted to attract African Americans but there was little interest in this practice.[8]

Obesity is at an all-time high among many different age, race, gender, and ethnic groups. Yoga cannot but help in this regard. Research suggests that greater body awareness, which is associated with greater body satisfaction and lower rates of eating disorders, is related to yoga practice. The absence of people of color on *YJ*'s covers speaks to the privileging of practice to white culture and raises important questions about the intent of yoga and its positioning as an option available only to particular communities. This seems contrary to the yogic philosophy. Furthermore, despite the fact that seventy-three percent of those who attend yoga classes are women, *YJ* would be doing a service by reaching out to men and those marketers who also sell yoga-related products for men.

Studies of young people's feelings about their bodies are finding yoga to be an important source of empowerment. Regardless of intensity or structure, the underlying philosophy espouses relief from individual and global suffering, liberation from limited ideas about ourselves and others, and concretized ways of thinking about the world. Yoga also promotes the development of moral principles of compassion and awareness, and the replacement of static with more fluid notions of self and others. Besides the salvation aspect of much Indian thought, self-awareness and

DEBRA MERSKIN

consciousness about one's role in alleviating the suffering of others is a tenet of yogic practice. While yoga's origins 'sprang from the soil of India,' yoga is understood as 'a liberation tradition for *all* humanity.'[9] Bound by neither time nor place, yoga's appeal is designed to stretch across cultures and economies, and, in that sense, according to Iyengar, 'it is a *radical* teaching which goes to the root (radix) of the problem: lethargy, fear of change, prejudice, self-delusion – all of which can be summarized as ignorance (*avidya*). The whole purpose of Yoga is to remove ignorance.'[10] Thus, I argue, the visual representation of a mind–body integrative practice such as yoga, in a publication such as *Yoga Journal*, bears special responsibility for presenting realistic and inclusive images on the cover.

NOTES

1   Julia Roberts, quoted in Anne Cushman, 'Americanized yoga: Is yoga losing its spirit by becoming mainstream?' *Yoga Journal* (January–February 2000, http://www.beliefnet.com/Holistic-Living/Yoga/How-To-Yoga/Americanized-Yoga.aspx#ixzz1EBZSyu7R).

2   Ian Brown, 'Is yoga getting bent out of shape?' *The Globe and Mail* (May 12, 2007), F1.

3   Dayna Macy, '*Yoga Journal* releases 2008 "yoga in America" market study,' *Yoga Journal* (February 26, 2008, http://www.yogajournal.com/advertise/press_releases/10).

4   'The *Yoga Journal* story' (n.d., http://yogajournal.com).

5   Erving Goffman, *Gender Advertisements* (New York: Harper & Row, 1979).

6   Steve Taylor, *100 Years of Magazine Covers* (London: Black Dog Publishing, 2006), p. 117.

7   T. K. V. Desikachar, *The Heart of Yoga: Developing a Personal Practice* (Rochester, VT: Inner Traditions, 1995), p. 23.

8   Maya Breuer, 'Yoga & African Americans' (UCLA Center for Communications & Community, n.d., http://www.c3.ucla.edu/research-reports/community-voice/yoga-and-african-americans).

9   B. K. S. Iyengar, *Light on Life* (New York: Rodale, 2006), p. xiv.

10 Ibid., p. 14.

PART 3

PRANA: YOGA'S VITAL ENERGY

CHAPTER 11

MY GUIDANCE COUNSELOR ALWAYS SAID I'D BE A GREAT YOGA STUDENT

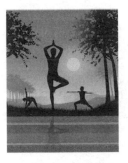

Most of us stumble upon yoga – through a friend or through our own curiosity – sometime in adulthood. It is not something we grow up practicing or knowing much about, much like meditation or, say, philosophy. We may see people stretching or hear the occasional adult claim that it changed his or her life, yet, because yoga is for the most part absent in our educational upbringing, we either never learn it or are led to believe we don't need it in the 'real world' – that is, until we're older and we discover we need health and relaxation to virtually save our lives. 'It's not like yoga can help you succeed in the world like math or reading can,' we can imagine our teachers saying when asked to explain the omission. And yet, once we encounter a good instructor and experience firsthand the rewards of intensive practice, we find ourselves reflecting, *if only I'd known about this earlier! I could have really used this!* What if our introduction to yoga wasn't by chance, but instead was part of a deliberate and comprehensive program to equip us with knowledge and skills for life? What if yoga were taught to children, as part of the educational curriculum in the public schools?

Yoga – Philosophy for Everyone: Bending Mind and Body, First Edition.
Edited by Liz Stillwaggon Swan.
© 2012 John Wiley & Sons, Inc. Published 2012 by John Wiley & Sons, Inc.

This essay explores the role that yoga can play in shaping the personal and social development of children. I draw upon my experience as both school counselor and yogi in order to explore how yoga can be used to help one's child, one's self, and one's students. I present various ways yoga can be used in a school setting in hopes that it will become an essential component of primary and secondary education, thus empowering students with a means for health and growth across the lifespan.

Looking Back

As one of fifteen million people practicing yoga in the United States today, I have directly experienced the benefits of yoga and count myself among those who wish they had learned yoga at a younger age. Sure, it would be great to have perfect form at age thirty-six as a result of having learned yoga while I was in elementary school, but, more importantly, I could have benefited from the personal and social development that emerges from regular yoga practice; after all, knowledge and skills last much longer than a toned physique! If I had learned through yoga how to 'go inward' and act with intention – aligning mind and body – I would have made decisions differently *then* and through the years that followed. Allow me to speculate on how this simple instruction alone could have helped shape my development.

Fundamentally, my decisions would have been more mindful, which is to say, in accordance with my 'innermost voice' – the voice that speaks with self-awareness, clarity, and sensitivity to others. Presumably, mindful choices would have led to the attainment of goals and personal achievement, friendships, and harmonious relationships, and would have buffered me from negative peer pressure – key factors for growth in childhood and adolescence. Moreover, I would argue that making good decisions bolsters self-esteem, which in turn increases self-confidence and bolsters self-concept (i.e., how we see ourselves). Thus, it is easy to imagine myself acting more purposefully and mindfully in the years following my being introduced to yoga, earning higher grades in high school and college, feeling good about my choices and who I was as a person – in large part because a yoga instructor taught me to slow down, focus, and demonstrate good form *off* the mat as well as on it.

I can't say with any certainty, but I believe the extent to which yoga would have helped shape my development would depend on the age at which I had been introduced to it. I suspect that the sooner I started 'stretching' my body and mind and learned to practice yoga as a means for health and wellness, self-discipline, and growth, the greater the impact would have been on my personal and social development. Knowledge and skills affect choices and their consequences in exponential ways; a simple insight can catapult you forward. Conversely, the lack of insight can inhibit growth or lead to 'arrested development.' It can cause you to make the same mistake over and over.

If you haven't done so already, take a moment and ask yourself: What if I had learned yoga as a child, during my elementary or middle school years? How might I be different today as a result?

Looking Forward

While we will never know how yoga could have changed our lives, personal experience tells us that stretching – body and mind – is inherently good for us. It's relaxing, restorative, and yet *invigorating*. It results in changes in mind and behavior – growth, at its essence. Research tells us that yoga fosters self-control, attention and concentration, body awareness, stress reduction, and self-efficacy (i.e., your belief in your ability to reach a goal). Additional research suggests that yoga is associated with increases in physical functioning and cardiovascular health. For these reasons, isn't it time adults made a push to promote yoga for children?

Before you answer that question, it might help to have more facts about how yoga is taught to kids as opposed to adults. Being curious myself, I found it helpful to read 'Yoga for children,' by Laura Santegelo White (2009). White investigates the subject from a clinical point of view and provides a concise summary of yoga philosophy, the different types of yoga, the necessary components of yoga programs for children, as well as resources and links for further inquiry. I learned that typical practice with children involves the same basic phases as yoga for adults: warm-up, breathing, posture work, and relaxation. In short, White writes, 'The focus in childhood is less on the perfection of postures than the cultivation of compassion, non-judgment, connection between breath and postures, and forging the foundations of a life-long practice.'[1] Until recently, I didn't think much about kids learning yoga. Then I met 'Harlow,' who convinced me that you're never too young to learn yoga.

Namaste

'How cool!' I thought, upon hearing that my friend's seven-year-old daughter is learning yoga at her elementary school, where she's a second-grader. For the modest price of sixty dollars, Harlow will receive six sessions, each an hour long, taught by a certified yoga instructor. My friend has never practiced yoga before and yet both he and the school administration are encouraging yoga; or, at the very least, yoga is being presented as an option, just like after-school soccer and basketball. For this to be the case, the adults must see the potential of yoga to nourish child development on some level, whether physical, social, psychological, or some combination of these. Maybe the adults in this school community see the value in exposing kids to yoga as a non-competitive, lighthearted activity – an antidote to the rigors of the school day – or, then again, maybe the allure of seeing a dozen elementary school kids in tree pose is simply too cute to deny.

When I asked Harlow what yoga meant to her she said, 'The light in me sees the light in you.' Her answer jolted me. Not bad for a seven-year-old! Some of you know that this is (roughly) the translation of 'namaste,' the greeting that typically begins and concludes a yoga practice. Others of you might say it sounds like Harlow is expressing something deeper, which I'll call 'respect for self and others.' It seems to me that both are true. What's important to consider here is that respect for self and others is a value that every parent wants to instill in his or her child and that every classroom teacher attempts to instill in his or her students – often with mixed results – and that this seven-year-old girl 'got' through yoga. I suspect that it will not be long before Harlow can articulate how each person (including herself) has his or her own beauty, special skill, right to live, and inner wisdom. Respect, compassion, tolerance – if nothing else, a simple *namaste* – has much to teach a developing child about living in the world.

From the Individual to the Universal

It is not just my friend and Harlow's particular school that are introducing kids to yoga. There is a whole new generation of adults, myself included, who have practiced yoga and want to share their discovery, especially with parents and leaders in educational reform, in the hope that yoga will become more visible and available to children. By now, we have all seen, perhaps both first-hand and in others, the consequences of stress and poor physical health and we should aim to instill healthier habits in children, in part by introducing them to yoga. The timing couldn't be better. Now more than ever, parents and educators across the United States are interested in education that extends beyond content and teaches students how to live and thrive. There seems to be greater concern for the 'whole' child these days, instead of just grades. Adults know firsthand how complex and challenging the world is; they know that a balance of 'hard' (i.e., academic, technical) and 'soft' (i.e., social, emotional) skills is necessary to succeed in college, the workplace, relationships – in life in general. Yoga, which is certainly known to improve one's sense of balance, literally and figuratively, has much to offer in the area of 'soft' skills.

What excites me the most about kids learning yoga is that a whole new generation will grow up equipped with a rather simple strategy – a tool – for cultivating health and wellness. Theoretically and realistically speaking, yoga practice can and will foster personal and social development, which is ever more valuable in an age of childhood obesity, teen depression and suicide, and bullying in schools. By teaching kids how to discipline their bodies and minds through *asana* (the physical poses) and *pranayama* (regulated breathing) practices, kids will develop mind–body coordination, self-discipline, and a heightened sense of focus, all of which can positively shape their outlook, choices, and behavior. As kids develop a greater awareness of their own bodies, feelings, and thoughts, they also develop a greater regard for the same in others. Empathy and compassion are the bases for peaceful relationships; developing a clear sense of these values early in life should facilitate 'success' throughout childhood, adolescence, and adulthood in school, work, and personal relationships.

Imagine a positive 'feedback loop' in which the more physically and mentally 'in tune' the child becomes, the better able he may be to approach peers and make friends; thus, he feels more liked, develops a better self-image, further engages in the world, and experiences personal and social growth. For some kids, a simple tool like yoga can make all the difference; it could literally change their lives. An anxious or shy child can easily benefit from the various relaxation and strengthening exercises taught in yoga. Literally and figuratively, kids learn to 'stretch instead of contract' in the face of life. In this way, their yoga practice extends beyond the mat and results in knowledge and skills for life. Experiential learning is a powerful teacher, and one of the most compelling aspects of yoga is that it allows you to witness your progress directly.

Consider how yoga might help kids develop better attention and concentration skills, including those who suffer from attention deficit disorder (ADD) or attention deficit hyperactivity disorder (ADHD). Session by session, for extended periods of time (sixty to ninety minutes, the length of a typical practice), kids could learn how to harness the power of self-control and concentration. Mentally, they would notice improvements in their listening skills and sense of focus, and physically they would notice improvements in their form (e.g., 'My triangle pose is getting stronger'). Visible, self-verifiable progress combined with positive teacher feedback increases one's self-efficacy ('I *can* do this'). Again, such skill acquisition could have significant personal and social implications; by curbing maladaptive behaviors, such as impulsivity and distractibility, a succession of positive changes could result, including increased self-esteem, peer acceptance, and success in school. Parents who are reluctant to medicate their children for ADD/ADHD might be interested in yoga as an alternative therapy.

Yoga in Schools

I graduated from high school in 1992 and have no memory of ever having heard the word 'yoga,' despite years of physical education (PE) and health classes, and after-school sports. You can consider yourself fortunate if yoga was taught in your public school system. In retrospect, it's disappointing to think that I attended 'strong' schools in suburban Connecticut where parents were educated and health-conscious, and athletic programs were well-funded, and yet yoga totally escaped mention. One might argue that in the 1980s and early 1990s yoga was still an untapped well, studios were scarce, and I'd accept that – this was, after all, the 'dark age' before you could 'tweet' and 'blog' about your discoveries for the world to seize upon. Few in the West had much exposure to yoga and, if they did, they were not necessarily involved in developing and implementing educational curricula.

But now we can expect that students will graduate from high school at least having been exposed to yoga through general PE classes, acquiring basic knowledge of the *asanas* and how they can be used for physical fitness and health. This could be done at any grade level; the earlier the better. We can also imagine opportunities for students to study yoga intensively, particularly at the high school level, when students could choose yoga for their PE elective, as an alternative to weight training or swimming. Perhaps levels of yoga could be offered, for example beginners' and intermediate. Such classes could inspire students to study yoga further, perhaps as a career or as a cross-training activity. Some schools – the more progressive and well-funded ones – have already adopted such measures in order to meet the needs of students, and perhaps to broaden their appeal to 'school-shopping' parents.

If you Google 'yoga in public schools' you can expect to find around fifteen million results. Clearly people are curious about the subject, and certainly there is varying public opinion. Advocates argue that yoga has the potential to increase students' physical fitness and enhance health and well-being. They support yoga's inclusion in schools, which is generally through PE classes. Opponents argue that yoga is a spiritual discipline and should not be practiced in school. They present their objections to school officials (and the media), refuse to have their children participate in yoga, and, in some cases, threaten to home-school their children out of defiance. Then there are those who have simply never thought much about it, but, if given a compelling argument and some evidence, might rally behind the cause. They'll start asking schools whether they offer it, and, if not, demand why not. In my experience as a school counselor for the last ten years, I have found that, when parents start advocating for their children, the system responds and change occurs for the better.

Furthering the Case for Yoga in Schools

In my career as a school counselor, it was not until recently that I saw a connection between yoga and part of my job description, namely my responsibility for leading activities that foster students' personal and social development. I knew that yoga nourished me and many others, but I was content to leave the job of introducing yoga to parents, or, in a school setting, to PE teachers. No counselors that I knew of were discussing yoga for students to any significant extent, and I certainly didn't have any science or case studies to support what I intuited, which was: yoga can nurture students' personal and social development as well as lead to academic achievement.

Having discovered Laura Santegelo White 'Yoga for children' article and the website www.yogaed.com in the course of writing this essay, I can now share data and research with my colleagues and administrative team in order to win their support for introducing yoga to students. For instance, studies have already investigated yoga in the context of academic performance and found a host of appealing outcomes, such as: increased IQ and social adaptation, increased academic achievement, improved decision-making skills, improved communication skills, and increased attention span.[2] These data make it much easier for me to present the case that yoga can have tangible benefits to students, and in turn the school itself, which can expect improvements in classroom behavior and test scores.

Keeping in mind the American School Counselor Association's (ASCA) Model (the framework governing my profession and the standards to which I am accountable), research supporting the educational uses of yoga allows me advocate for yoga as a means for student achievement (Domain One) and personal and social development (Domain Three). This is exciting for those of us who hope to see yoga in schools because a case can be made by other counselors too that yoga has a place in public education. The more that counselors and the education community learn about the benefits of yoga and, more importantly, give voice to those benefits, the more likely it is that schools and parents will support yoga as essential curriculum.

Specific, Additional Options Worth Considering

There are many ways to include yoga in education and one way of looking at the spectrum of possibilities is to consider levels of implementation: there are the individual, the group, the building, and eventually the school system 'levels.' Depending on your comfort zone, level of expertise, and degree of support from your principal, you can incorporate yoga accordingly. Based on my own situation, here are a few things I would hope to add to my work with students. For the sake of simplicity, these strategies could be used with students of all grade levels, unless mentioned otherwise.

On the individual level, I would teach simple deep breathing exercises to students who suffer from anxiety, panic attacks, or stress – most likely after discussing the intent and viability of this strategy with the parent(s).

To impulsive students with attention problems, I would introduce 'quieting the mind' as a means for self-discipline, self-awareness, and getting along better with classmates. Sometimes kids are simply *unaware* of how their natural state of being affects others; students could be taught to notice how an irritating behavior is perceived by classmates and learn to self-correct. When counseling students who are seeking change, I would present yoga as a means for 'stretching' outside their comfort zones. It's a perfect metaphor and practice for achieving slow but steady growth; oftentimes a little stretching and meditation can guide you toward your own 'answers.' Finally, I would use yoga with kids suffering from low self-esteem and self-efficacy. Even a kid who 'can't do anything right' can do a powerful warrior pose and in turn feel empowered.

On a group level, I would like to discuss with students the ways that yoga could facilitate personal and social development. I would present yoga as a self-care strategy for facilitating exercise, alignment, relaxation, and stress-busting. Counselors often lead such discussions – or, as we call them, 'developmental classroom guidance lessons.' I see the merit in teaching a specific *asana* to a group of students in order to illustrate a point, such as aligning body and mind in order to focus, make good choices, and reach goals. I can also imagine myself, and most other counselors for that matter, incorporating an *asana* or two into a group counseling setting, such as an anger management or self-esteem group. The use of guided relaxation or a visualization exercise could give kids the necessary cognitive framework to facilitate behavioral change. You could easily also teach this in a classroom, since students respond very well to calming, stress-busting activities. Surely teachers could find a use for 'quiet time' that serves students, such as after recess, before a test, or as part of any 'brainstorming' activity.

On a building level, three main ideas come to mind. One, the possibility of incorporating comprehensive and sequential curriculum, either developed by the counselor(s) or a third party, such as Yoga Ed.[3] This curriculum, as developed by Tara Gruber, sounds extremely promising; it spans pre-kindergarten through grade twelve, it meets state and national physical education standards, it develops self-awareness and life skills, it lays a foundation for lifetime health and wellness – *and* there are compelling research and testimonials affirming its effectiveness and benefits to students. I wish I had known about this curriculum earlier! Two, I would encourage the PE department at my school to include yoga in their curriculum (if they were not already), and, at the high school level, I would advocate for beginner and intermediate yoga classes. And finally – sorry kids, this one's for adults – I would love to provide a yoga class for staff, who work so hard and accumulate so much stress, which often inadvertently affects the students. I have found that principals (and counselors) enjoy giving back to their staff, and funding a couple of yoga sessions to be held after school or during 'professional development' time would be well worth the money. It's amazing what staff will do when they feel personally cared for and valued.

Conclusion

Surely, yoga has the potential to foster personal and social development in kids as well as adults. It is high time we took the risk as educators, parents, yogis, and yoginis and advocated for yoga to be considered essential learning – knowledge and skills for life. It is my hope that yoga will find a permanent place in primary and secondary education and become integrated into the curriculum. In an era of significant school reform, when educational leaders such as Michelle Rhee are seeking ways to completely transform school systems, I hope that yoga will be mentioned in the discussion about what's good for kids. One day, when these kids are adults, they will be grateful for having been given such a valuable tool, a tool that served them well throughout their most challenging years. *Namaste.*

NOTES

1   Laura Santegelo White, 'Yoga for children,' *Pediatric Nursing* (2009, Vol. 35, No.5), p. 279.
2   'Research and assessments' (n.d., http://www.yogaed.com).
3   http://www.yogaed.com.

CHAPTER 12

BALANCE IN YOGA AND ARISTOTLE[1]

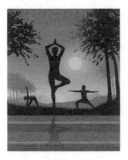

At a certain point in my studies as a graduate student, I found myself stressed out, overworked, and exhausted. I put so much importance on doing well academically that I neglected other aspects of my life. Having such a regimented lifestyle, I made no room for family, friends, or even yoga. The stress manifested itself physically: I collapsed in public, spent three days in a hospital, and was finally told that I had had a stress-induced grand-mal seizure. Something had to change. I tried returning to my yoga practice, but even on the mat my type-A personality took over. I often found myself pushing too hard to get into a pose that was not right for me. I would try too hard and end up holding my breath – a key sign that one is not really practicing yoga.

My teacher encouraged the class to find balance – not just a physical balance in each pose but a balance between strength and ease. How can we challenge ourselves, yet not push to the point of pain? She then related this lesson to our lives off our mats, asking whether we have balance there. Do we try too hard and wear ourselves out or do we not

Yoga – Philosophy for Everyone: Bending Mind and Body, First Edition.
Edited by Liz Stillwaggon Swan.
© 2012 John Wiley & Sons, Inc. Published 2012 by John Wiley & Sons, Inc.

try enough? Do we dare to do too much or do we never dare to do what we are actually able to do? I immediately recognized myself in the former group. My exhaustion and stress were results of pushing myself too hard and not balancing strength and determination with ease and comfort.

At the same time, I was teaching the Nichomachean ethics to an undergraduate class and discussing Aristotle's views on how to live a good life. As I explained the Aristotelian idea of the 'mean' to the class, it occurred to me that this was very similar to the idea of balance my yoga teacher had been talking about. For Aristotle, in order to be good, we must cultivate the virtues; each of the virtues is an intermediary between a deficiency and an excess. Tending toward an excess of work and study, I was missing the intermediary or the balance between work and relaxation, between pushing myself to do better and being kind to myself in times of stress. Thinking about how both of these teachings were applicable to my own life, I began to see how much the teachings of yoga have in common with the teachings of Aristotle. Both emphasize the importance of balance in our lives and, for both, this balance is relative to the individual. The 'right' pose in yoga depends on the individual and his or her body. The mean for Aristotle also depends on the individual and his or her strengths and weaknesses.

Balance and the Mean

Balance is essential to yoga. Even in a pose such as *samasthiti* (basic standing pose), we must find balance to connect to the ground. We lean into our toes and then into our heels in order to disrupt that balance so that we can start anew and equally distribute our weight in all corners of our feet. As we move into more complex poses or ones that are specifically balancing poses, this sense of balance may become a little more difficult to find or a little more important to achieve in order to hold the pose. For example, in *vrksasana* (tree pose), we balance on the standing foot to remain upright. In *bakasana* (crow pose), we balance on our hands so we don't fall forward. However, balance is key to not only individual *asanas* but the entire practice of yoga. Throughout the physical practice, we aim to cultivate a balance of two yogic qualities: *sthira* and *sukha*.

Loosely translated, '*sthira*' refers to a sense of strength. It is the quality required to hold a difficult lunge or a challenging arm balance. It is also sometimes translated as 'steadiness,' 'stability,' or 'alertness.' It allows us to endure challenges and to stand firm, connecting with the ground beneath us. It keeps our minds focused when they wander. '*Sukha*' refers to ease or openness. It is the quality required to open our heart centers and expand our upper bodies in *virabhadrasana* I (warrior I). It keeps the pose buoyant with lightness. It is also sometimes translated as 'pleasantness,' 'comfort,' 'happiness,' or 'relaxation.' It is the opposite of discomfort and pain. It is a sense of being light and comfortable in the pose.

In the *Yoga Sutras* (11.46), Patañjali says '*sthira sukha*m *asanam*': '*asana* is a perfect firmness of body, steadiness of intelligence and benevolence of spirit.'[2] Here, Patañjali emphasizes the importance of both qualities in *asana*. The firmness of the body is essential to hold the pose, but the benevolence of the spirit is essential for yoga. Yoga, after all, is a union of body, breath, mind, and spirit. In order for the body to unite with the mind, the mind cannot be caught up in the struggle of holding the pose. However, if the mind is too light and unfocused, the pose may not reach its full potential and the yoga is lost. There must be lightness to the pose, *sukha*, as well as strength, *sthira*.

For example, I will probably never be able to do *svarga dvijasana* (bird of paradise pose). My hamstrings might never be open enough for me to raise my foot above my shoulder and my spinal cord might not ever be straight enough for me to stand all the way up. But I have seen able yoga teachers in very beautiful full versions of the pose. These same yoga teachers encourage me to at least try some version of the pose and to find ease in whatever version that is right for me. Can I lift my foot just slightly off the ground? Through my breath, can I rise just a bit more each time I rediscover the pose? This is *sthira*. It is the ability to breathe through the struggle. I shake, my hamstring burns, and, though I want to come out of the pose, I find strength to hold it because I can. *Sthira* allows me to do what I am able even when I don't believe that I am able.

If, conversely, I were to push too hard, I could tear my hamstring or dislocate my shoulder. In yoga, we need to be aware of the difference between discomfort and pain. The discomfort I may feel in *virabhadrasana* I is nothing like the pain I might feel if I tried to push myself into a full *svarga dvijasana*. I know my hamstrings are not flexible enough to be in the full version of the pose. To try and force it is to not respect my limitations. *Sthira* does not require me to push myself beyond my limits but to test the limits I *think* I have. *Sthira* allows me to find that the threshold is just a little past where I thought it was. It is the courage to go a little deeper and to challenge myself to hold the pose a little longer.

Once I have found that strength, I must then find the ability to relax in the pose. Holding either *virabhadrasana* I or my own version of *svarga dvijasana* is challenging. The question is whether I can find some ease within that challenge and whether I can allow my heart center to open. This is *sukha*. Through the discomfort, through the struggle, I try to find a lightness and I do so through my breath. While in a deep lunge in *virabhadrasana* I, my thighs tire, my shoulders ache, and I wonder how much longer I must hold the pose. But, as I take a few deep, focused breaths, I relax into the pose. I do not collapse into it though: my knee stays centered over my toes and my arms reach skyward – but I no longer struggle. I unclench my jaw and relax my shoulders down from my ears so that my heart can open. This is *sukha*. Within the challenge – and all the while using *sthira* to hold the pose – I have *sukha*. I find ease within the challenge and a buoyancy of spirit as I enjoy the yoga. It is this balance of qualities that allows each yogi to come into his or her own personal best version of a pose in that particular moment.

Balance is also key to understanding the Aristotelian idea of living a good and virtuous life. In the *Nichomachean Ethics*, Aristotle says, 'Excellence then, is a state concerned with choice, lying in a mean relative to us, this being determined by reason and in the way in which the man of practical wisdom would determine it.'[3] While each part of this quote is important to understanding Aristotle's ethics, it is the idea of a mean relative to us that is so similar to the idea of individual balance we find in yoga. The mean, an intermediary between two extremes, is very much like the right balance between *sthira* and *sukha*.

For Aristotle, the virtues are not an intermediary between two *actions*, but are better thought of as an intermediary between two types of personality traits. For example, one of the virtues Aristotle discusses is courage. To be a courageous person, one does not need to act courageously in each and every dangerous situation. The courageous person knows when it is appropriate to act in the face of danger and when it is not. A person who avoids all dangerous or scary situations is called a coward. This is the deficit of the virtue. Conversely, it is not always right to act in the face of danger. Sometimes, acting in such a situation would cause more harm than good since sometimes we are limited in what we can do. In those cases, acting would not be courageous but instead would be foolish and rash. This is the excess. A courageous person finds the balance between the two extremes in the mean.

Another virtue Aristotle discusses is good temper. This refers to being angry in the right situations at the right time and for the right reasons.

In having a good temper, a person expresses anger at injustices. This virtue is supposed to incite us to act so that we can change the situation for the better. However, it is important not to act angrily *any* time one feels angry. We would call such a person irascible; this is the excess. If you become angry when someone cuts you off in traffic, it would be inappropriate to express that anger. It does no good. There is no great injustice to remedy and, moreover, acting angrily while still driving is dangerous for the driver and everyone else on the road. However, it's just as important to express anger when appropriate. If you become angry because you have witnessed a large group of teenagers bullying a younger and helpless child, it would be appropriate to act out of anger in order to help the child. To have a good temper, one must know when it is appropriate to be angry and when it is not.

In order to have this particular virtue of good temper, we need *sthira*. We need the strength to stand up for what is right and just, to stand up for our principles. We need focus to remember what those principles are and to not be swayed by popular opinion. At the same time, having a *good* temper is not acting on any and every feeling of anger. Good temper is purposeful and it manifests itself in actions that are intended to change an injustice. We also need *sukha*. We need that quality of ease to remain calm when a situation may make us angry but when it would be inappropriate to act out of anger. We need to keep an open heart so that we are not acting angrily to someone who does not deserve to feel our wrath. The open heart can allow you to recognize that the person who cut you off in traffic may not have seen you or may have been rushing home to a sick child. In being open, we can keep perspective so that we only act out of anger when it is really virtuous to do so.

Individuality

Sthira and *sukha* are like the extremes of the Aristotelian virtues. Just as it is sometimes right to act and be courageous and it is sometimes right to hold yourself back, sometimes it is right to challenge yourself to go a little deeper in a pose and sometimes it is better to ease off. But what is 'right' depends on the individual and the moment. This is true for the Aristotelian virtues and for our yoga practice. The right amount of *sthira* and the right amount of *sukha* depend on the individual yogi, his or her body and practice that day, and the pose. For example, poses such as *svarga dvijasana* are challenging for a person who prefers restorative poses and require that person to find more *sthira*. But poses such as rag doll require more letting go and might prove challenging for a person who approaches the pose without *sukha*. Just as it is sometimes very difficult to find the *sthira* to hold a challenging lunge, sometimes it is just as difficult to surrender into a deep forward fold. *Sukha* helps us let go.

The right balance also depends on the individual. The right version of *virabhadrasana* I will look different depending on the individual's body. The lunge shouldn't be as deep for my father, who has had two hips replaced, as it is for me. I have tight hamstrings, but I also have very open hip flexors. I can hold a pretty deep lunge in *virabhadrasana* I on my good days, and on those days a deep lunge is right for me. But, the right version of *virabhadrasana* I for me on one day is not the same as it is on any other given day. The right balance of *sthira* and *sukha* also depends on my body in that moment. In the days after finishing my first half-marathon, I needed to back out of the lunge a bit since my legs were recovering.

Finally, the right balance of *sthira* and *sukha* also depends on individual temperaments. I tend to push too much and so, after the race, I needed to focus on relaxation and enjoying yoga through *sukha*. I have a good friend who tends to lack focus; even during her practice, her mind wanders to all the other things going on in her life. Her work is in staying present through *sthira*. Then there is the person new to yoga who believes that yoga is merely about relaxing and is surprised when he is actually physically challenged in his first class. His work is to dare to do more than just stretch in sitting poses. He needs to be reminded that he too has an edge and can work at that edge without injury or pain.

The individual nature of balance is part of Aristotle's theory too. Aristotle says,

> fear and confidence and appetite and anger and pity and in general pleasure and pain may be felt both too much and too little, and in both cases not well; but to feel them at the right times, with reference to the right objects, towards the right people, with the right aim, and in the right way, is what is both intermediate and best, and this is characteristic of excellence.[4]

The virtues are a mean 'relative to us.' As Aristotle points out, in certain cases in which it is appropriate for a soldier to act in the face of danger, it is not appropriate for an elder to act. However, it might not always be appropriate for the soldier to act either. If his very life would be in danger, it might be better for him to step back. While he needs strength to act in the face of danger, he also needs to be aware of his own limitations *and* to be able to accept them. To be generous, another virtue, is to give the right amount, at the right time, and to the right people. But what is 'right' depends on the generous person's individual circumstances. What is right for Bill Gates is not right for the struggling college student! Still, both can be generous by finding the mean relative to their individual circumstances.

Aristotle says that, in choosing to act virtuously, we do so for the sake of 'kalon' – the beautiful, noble, or fine. In practicing yoga with a balance of *sthira* and *sukha*, we strive for that same ideal. *Sthira* in our physical practice is strength in the right time, for the right pose, and with the right aim – the aim being yoga, not looking a certain way in the pose. *Sukha* is ease in the right time, for the right pose, and with the right aim – the aim, again, being yoga, not avoiding any struggle whatsoever. We should not be so eager to get into the most difficult of poses, yet we should not be afraid to try something that is really within our capabilities. The correct balance of *sthira* and *sukha*, 'correct' for the individual, will form a state of *satva* – equilibrium – or, in Aristotle's words, a mean.

In order to know what is right for you in your physical yoga practice or in cultivating the virtues, you must know yourself and be honest with yourself about your strengths and limitations. Honesty and truthfulness to self also happen to be Aristotelian virtues. Before my seizure, I exaggerated my strengths, an excess that Aristotle calls 'boastfulness.' I did this in my physical yoga practice and in my daily life. I was overly confident and didn't ask for help when I really needed it. I did not recognize my own limitations and I tried to do too much. What I needed was to find the intermediary of humility and pride in order to recognize what I was unable to do. My personality often calls for more *sukha*; my challenge is to learn to back off and be kind to myself. Others need more *sthira*. I have a relative who tends to understate her strengths and needs more *sthira*. She has been in the same position at work for years even though she is very good at what she does. She could move up in her career if she had the proper confidence in herself and wasn't afraid to say, 'I am good at what I do. Promote me!'

Moving Off the Mat

There are many lessons from our physical yoga practice that can be beneficial in our lives off the mat, for example remembering to breathe and being present. Having balance is one of those lessons. Maintaining a balance between strength and ease can help us in all sorts of areas of our daily lives. When we are faced with an emotionally challenging situation, for example, we may need *sthira* to deal with it. We need the strength to try and make what changes we can, a firmness to stick to our beliefs, and courage to be responsible for our actions. We may also need *sukha*. We need ease to accept what we cannot change with grace, openness in order to go with the flow and deal with the challenge in a calm and peaceful way, and lightness to be kind to ourselves and to others.

Before the seizure, my life was very regimented. In order to do all that I thought I had to do, I set aside certain hours to work on my lesson plans, read for class, write, practice yoga, clean my house, do my laundry, and so on. I was overly firm with myself so that I would be a successful student, would be a good teacher, would have a clean house, would be physically fit, and so forth. I didn't make room for anything that didn't fit into the plan, including feeling upset when I didn't do as well academically as I expected to, or spending time with a good friend when she was having marital problems. I lacked *sukha*. My heart center was not open because I focused too much on being strong, focused, and steady. I tended toward the excess of pride and courage and never let myself be vulnerable when I should have.

A friend of mine lost his job as an accountant after years of being with one practice. He never really liked filing other people's taxes, though he loved discussing financial matters. He also happened to be a naturally talented teacher. In this case, by being honest with himself about his strengths and weaknesses, he realized that the best way to deal with his job loss was to switch career paths. He began teaching accounting classes at a local community college simply in order to make ends meet at first and discovered that he loved it. He could only do this by finding a balance of *sthira* and *sukha*. He had strength to risk changing careers *and* was kind to himself when he gave up on a career path that he had had for so long. In the Aristotelian sense, he was virtuous in knowing when it was right for him to act.

In the *asanas*, *sthira* connects us to the ground beneath us and *sukha* allows the heart to open. In life, these two yogic qualities have the same effects. *Sthira* grounds us. It keeps us focused and lets us think practically. It gives us strength to act. *Sukha* on the other hand lets us experience whatever emotions may arise. It is how we can open up to others and how we can be open to others. With the correct balance of both qualities, a person can at the same time be practical about what he can and cannot change and also allow himself to feel his emotions, recognize his limitations, and be open to possibilities. To live a good life, according to Aristotle, we need to find the proper balance in each of the virtues. We not only need the strength to act but also the intellectual virtue to realize when it is appropriate to do so. We need to be gentle with ourselves, but only when it is right to do so; sometimes it is better to be hard on ourselves in order to push ourselves toward the threshold that is right for us.

This lesson is applicable to many other situations in everyday life. To be a good parent, it is important to have *sthira* in order to have and enforce rules that keep children healthy and safe, but it is equally important to have *sukha* in order to be kind and loving as they grow and to be understanding of their individual needs. To be successful in our jobs, we need *sthira* to have focus and goals, but we need *sukha* to go with the flow when things are out of our control. To be good academics, we need to have *sthira* in order to focus on our goals and push ourselves to do well, but we need *sukha* to know when to back off and take some time to enjoy other things in life such as our friends, our families, or our yoga.

Conclusion: Lesson Learned

Having found this common lesson in yoga and in Aristotle's ethics allowed me to recognize the imbalance in my own life. I tended toward excesses. I was not kind to myself and did not allow myself to feel the stress in my life. I thought that practicing yoga would help, but, even there, I pushed myself so much that on certain days it was no longer yoga. I lost the connection with my breath, I focused too much on how the pose looked, and I worried if I couldn't get into a pose that I used to be able to do. By finding the balance of *sthira* and *sukha* that was correct for me and for different poses on different days, I found my yoga. I gained a sense of ease so that I could relax. In doing so, I could focus more on my breath and less on the look of the pose. I learned to be kind to myself and not push myself past my threshold. I allowed myself to relax in *shavasana* (corpse pose) and simply be present with my breath.

Connecting the yoga lesson of balance to the Aristotelian lesson of the mean, I discovered the sense of balance that was missing in my life off the mat. I stopped being so hard on myself in terms of my academic work. I learned to be more open to others and to graciously accept help. When I found my stress manifesting itself in places it shouldn't, I remembered to breathe and to relax. But I didn't slip into a complete life of ease either. I found strength and steadiness to focus on my work when I needed to do so. It was only with this appropriate balance that the work became the right kind of work for me. Now, by reminding myself of the value of balance or of the mean, I strive to become virtuous in all areas of my life: to be generous, courageous, and honest; and to have a *good* temper and *proper* pride. If we cultivate the Aristotelian virtues, we will know when it is right to act and when it is right to let go.

NOTES

1 For Darcy, who first taught me about *sthira* and *sukha*.
2 B. K. S. Iyengar, *Light on the Yoga Sutras of Patañjali* (India: Harper Collins, 1993), p. 149.
3 Aristotle, *Nichomachean Ethics*. In J. Barnes (Ed.), *The Complete Works of Aristotle* (Princeton, NJ: Princeton University Press, 1984), 1106b36–1107a2.
4 Ibid., 1106b19–23.

CHAPTER 13

HEALING THE WESTERN MIND THROUGH YOGA

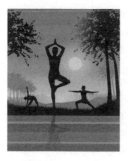

While it is well known that yoga practice has spiritual components, many newcomers find themselves on the mat for the first time in search of greater physical health or, at most, stress relief. They are often lucky to find something much greater: a holistic practice that increases the health of the whole person. Yoga is quickly becoming known not just for its physical health benefits and for giving one a sense of spirituality but also as a way to learn to manage one's mind. Students notice that, with consistent practice, shifts occur in their reactions to things both on and off the mat, resulting in a calmer, more centered, and more conscious way of carrying themselves.

Meanwhile, clinical studies are being conducted to test yoga's efficacy as an alternative or supplemental treatment for all kinds of mental illnesses – and the results are often positive. Doctors have long recommended physical activity as an important part of maintaining health, and now some psychologists and therapists are specifically recommending yoga to their clients. The yoga world is in a unique place – we as practitioners and teachers can choose how and when to work in conjunction with therapy. Most teachers and psychologists would agree that yoga cannot replace

Yoga – Philosophy for Everyone: Bending Mind and Body, First Edition.
Edited by Liz Stillwaggon Swan.
© 2012 John Wiley & Sons, Inc. Published 2012 by John Wiley & Sons, Inc.

psychotherapy for issues such as depression or stress; however, yoga teachers may have to understand how to step into the therapist's shoes from time to time.

In this essay, I will consider the intersection of yogic and psychological viewpoints on mental illness and what it means to be healthy. I will discuss some of the ways yoga can increase self-awareness, resiliency, relaxation, and quality of life. With that basis, I will look at some of the opportunities for professionals in both yoga and the mental health fields to strengthen or deepen their work with the minds and bodies of their students and clients.

Yoga's Approach to the Core Self

Yoga practitioners and mental health professionals have radically different ideas about the origins and nature of disease. Raja yoga metaphysics considers the self to be housed not just in a body but in a system of five interconnected sheaths. These range from the gross, or physical (the food and air that make up the corporeal body) to the subtle and energetic (mental processes, wisdom, and bliss). The important part of the sheaths for this essay is the idea of the bliss sheath inside all of the others, and the self even within that; that is, the belief that happiness and calmness are within at all times. Yoga distinguishes this true self from the ego, which identifies with likes and dislikes, aversions and experience, limiting concepts of self. The true inner self can never, by its nature, be unhealthy, and it is this self with which we seek to identify.

The body is also home to a network of energy channels, or *nadis*, that connect at several junctures or wheels called *chakras*. It is helpful to think of the *chakras* as energy centers – anatomical locations where a significant amount of physical processes as well as personal and cultural meanings converge. In traditional yogic thought, illness, disease, and stress are experiences of a blocked or distorted energy flow, while clear energy channels allow the true self to emerge. This 'true self' refers to the spark of universal life within each of us, a self that transcends our egos – our thoughts, preferences, and beliefs. A yogic lifestyle, which includes not only posture (*asana*) but also breath work (*pranayama*), meditation practices, and ethical lifestyle choices, is intended to purify these channels, encourage perception from the gross to the subtle sheaths, and foster discernment between the illusion of the ego and the bliss of reality.

ABBY THOMPSON

By learning to manage and regulate energy in this way, the yogi is free from suffering. Most Hatha yoga classes will not include a comprehensive education in yoga metaphysics, nor is this necessary to experience some of these benefits. Later in this essay, I will discuss some of the simple ways in which both teachers and therapists help the student or client to discern the truth in his or her experience and find a greater range of physical and emotional well-being.

Clinical Psychology and Treatment

The view of modern psychology is radically different to that of yoga, though the two paradigms are not mutually exclusive. The medical and psychology fields have, for the most part, established mental illness as a disruption in brain chemistry, cognition, and feeling, collectively. The *Diagnostic and Statistical Manual (DSM)* offers a systematized way to diagnose disorders. A diagnosis code from the *DSM* then allows therapists or psychologists to create an effective treatment plan, and allows the client or professional to bill the work to insurance companies. In some cases, this work involves the use of psychoactive medication, support groups, or other treatment strategies. While therapy and other treatments require a diagnosis, yoga is available to anyone, in increasingly diverse locations and settings that are outside of the healthcare and insurance system. Because it is useful as both prevention and coping, yoga has the potential to decrease the number of diagnoses and complications from existing illnesses.

In yoga, even if a particular problem emerges (e.g., fear of taking risks that manifests when attempting arm balances, or pain from an old injury), it does not become the focus of the practice. Even if the student takes his or her problem to a private lesson and asks the teacher to create a personalized practice around the concern, directly trying to undo the problem will only be a small part of the work. Yoga is always about developing and strengthening the whole person, creating ease and relaxation whether the pre-existing conditions are perfect for it or not. While talk therapy often works by finding strengths and releasing anxieties around the presenting problem rather than bluntly attacking it, the hope is that the problem will be solved and that the therapy session can end. Cognitive-behavioral therapy, for example, is often done on a very short-term basis – the problem is solved, coping skills are in place, and the client is sent on his or her way. Yoga can also facilitate solutions quickly and dramatically; but, if the student chooses, yoga can be a lifelong practice that spans many experiences, and endlessly deepens not just coping skills but the capacity to enjoy every moment.

How Yoga can Help

Cognitive-behavioral therapy is one of the most popular and effective talk therapy modalities available today. In addition to its measurable effect, it teaches frameworks for dealing with unpleasant emotions – 'teachable skills' that can be used outside the therapist's office. Yoga has been offering its own teachable skills passed down from guru to disciple, teacher to student, even DVD to living-room student, for thousands of years. To try this at home, think about a recent stressor. Really sit in that stress for a few seconds. Notice what sensations arise in the body, notice the breath. Now, bring all of your attention to your big toe. Notice if the edge has disappeared at all from that feeling of stress. Quickly scan your body for signs of that stress. This time, bring all of your attention to your breath as you take one long, smooth, deep belly breath and let it out just as smoothly. Check on that stress level again. Just by doing that, you may find that you are in a calmer, clearer state to deal with whatever the stressor might be. On the mat, in a pose such as *virabhadrasana* II (warrior II: see Figure 13.1), a student might be asked to draw attention to the outer edge of their left foot, kneecap, right thigh, pelvic floor, lower belly, shoulders, and fingertips (among other places) over the course of several slow, deep, conscious breaths. In this way, the student strengthens his or her ability to access and maintain that calm clarity even as his or her strength and flexibility improve. In addition, a comprehensive yoga education would also teach philosophical approaches to life on and off the mat, giving students a new framework in which to think about their problems.

As one notices gradual shifts in mood and physical well-being, one is more likely to be willing to see the ways in which yoga can be symbolic of one's general emotional life. Many schools of yoga have a simple aphorism that states, 'How you are on the mat is how you are in life.' This encourages a sense of self-care and reflection in thinking about and doing a posture practice. In yoga, we practice not only physical and emotional range and flexibility but also staying present with whatever

ABBY THOMPSON

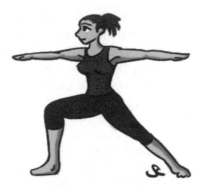

FIGURE 13.1 Warrior II. Thanks to Sharlene Leong of www.sparklydoom.com for the illustration.

emotional and physical experiences we are faced with. This practice of presence can extend to other aspects of our lives, especially relationships. By identifying, and not backing away, from discomfort, we allow ourselves the space to choose how we will respond to it. This can mean using that space to listen more carefully to a significant other or a child, or slowing down to recognize our underlying, less voiced needs.

Yoga practice, like life, is not at all devoid of discomfort. As a student develops mindfulness, he or she learns to distinguish between the pain signals that indicate one is doing harm to the body and the constructive discomfort that occurs when one is exercising outside of one's comfort level. This discernment allows the improving student to take on more advanced *asanas* or work on a deeper level in basic ones, and improves the experience of the overall practice. Pain is to be avoided so as not to incur injury, but a student can learn to manage discomfort to allow for rapid growth. A well-trained teacher will help show that the discomfort is not happening just on a physical level but is also happening on a metaphorical level; the student is developing a greater capacity to discern emotional pain from discomfort, allowing him or her to make better decisions in areas such as relationships or work. In the warrior II example, it might be sensing in the body and noticing that plenty of muscular pain in the front thigh can be endured, but not potentially injurious pain in the knee. With this awareness, the yoga student may be better able to decide when a relationship simply requires a difficult conversation, or is harmful to his or her well-being.

A parallel physical-metaphorical connection is that of alignment. While yoga schools vary greatly in the emphasis they place on aligning the body properly in poses, all schools include at least a basic understanding of the architecture of a pose. This is generally worked from the ground up, beginning with a steady base, followed by adjustments that deepen the stretch in a safe way. This step-by-step logic can be applied to personal problem-solving as well – it makes sense to have a solid grounding before pursuing other challenges. Only with a sense of solid grounding can alignment begin to work on muscle groups to ensure that particular muscles aren't overworking in the place of others – to make sure the overall effort works toward the desired effect of the *asana*. In warrior II, pressing evenly through all four corners of both feet steadies the legs so the thighs can work harder, and dropping the tailbone helps keep the spine straight.

Neuroscience and You

Posture is not just about how we hold ourselves upright; it has a lot to do with who we are. Recent developments in neuroscience, as well as the history of somatic psychology, have established that bodily habits – posture and movement, for example – are learned not just in parallel with the way thought patterns are established, but also in conjunction with ways of using the body. The mantra is, 'neurons that fire together, wire together,' meaning that the neuronal connections underlying our thoughts and feelings are strengthened every time they are elicited. For example, when someone learns from experience to tense her shoulders while feeling anxious, the neuronal activity in the brain that causes the sympathetic nervous system to activate (which is experienced as anxiety) becomes 'wired to' the neuronal activity that causes the shoulder-tension impulse. And, with repetition, the two become paired.

When we practice yoga, we practice different ways of being in our bodies, different pairings of physical shapes and emotional states. Sometimes, this means trying on new ways of holding ourselves up or letting ourselves relax, which naturally involves new ways of approaching things emotionally. We may be a warrior, with a strong, broad chest and active legs; a triangle, with a solid foundation; a plow, digging in; or a peacock, displaying our impressive strength and flexibility. Just like with the muscular tension, practicing these poses is literally 'practicing' these ways of being, giving us a greater range of physical and emotional expression. Alternatively, we can 'train' holding bodily stress while maintaining a sense of calm. Just as body shapes and thought patterns can 'train' together, like in the example of tight shoulders, we can gradually create a body and mind that are wired to be comfortable and at ease.

Getting Stronger, Getting Smarter

All of these converging practices and processes in yoga help us to develop a crucial skill – the ability to self-regulate. Response to sensation, feelings, and effort are all drawn out, and the task for the yogi is to maintain a calm mind, steady body, and deep breathing throughout the experience. And you thought it was just putting your foot behind your head! Like muscle strength, the ability to withstand these waves of psychological energy grows with practice. Yoga students often find themselves gradually less overwhelmed by stressors and difficulties, more emotionally flexible and strong, and able to connect to an internal sense of calm. Students also learn how to use body position and breathing style throughout their daily lives to increase their energy levels, maintain focus, and self-soothe.

When we begin to listen to signals from our bodies, we often find pain and discomfort first. Learning how to deal with these is a great first step toward resiliency and health. But, if yoga were all about tapping into the pain we all carry around, it would never have become as popular as it is. In yoga, we learn to find pleasure in our bodily experience too, and, when it appears, it often opens us to enjoying the practice more dramatically. Returning to our warrior II example, even with aching shoulders, the sense of expansiveness across the chest as the collarbones spread can be enormously satisfying. In the typical contemporary sedentary lifestyle, we generally expect bodily pleasure from eating, sex, and sleeping – and maybe not much else. So, finding joy in movement can be a radical experience for some. Because warrior II involves an extension in all directions, it can also create an enjoyable experience of expansiveness and taking up space – something one might not expect to like if one originally came to yoga to help manage weight. Off the mat, the experience of feeling comfortable and capable in one's own body can be profound.

Pain experiences, when we learn to tolerate and prevent them sensitively, can actually lead to more enjoyment as well. For example, the piriformis muscle that covers the major nerve in the outer hips releases resistance after a minute of gentle stretching, so holding a passive stretch such as half pigeon for a few minutes can help someone have the experience of initial discomfort tangibly dissolving into relaxation. Metaphorically, we can look at the sources of pain in our lives and look for where they help us open up to find new sources of pleasure, good feelings, or relationships.

Instructor Responsibility

As we begin to recognize yoga as a way to enhance mental well-being, instructors begin to have greater responsibility. A standard 200-hour Yoga Alliance teacher training course, which is required to teach and purchase insurance for most classes, involves some anatomy training to prevent injuries and modify the practice for existing conditions. But the same level of care needs to be given to the emotional well-being of students. Instructors need to be aware that pushing someone to the edge of his strength or stamina may also push him to an emotional edge; that physically vulnerable poses may evoke memories of vulnerable situations; and that, in general, people may be more fragile on the mat than in other situations. For example, a backbend such as *ustrasana* (camel pose) greatly exposes the heart and belly, which people, especially women, often keep protected with rounded shoulders and spines. The student may understandably feel exposed. Other students may feel vulnerable or unsteady when confronted with the limitations of their strength or balance. This creates many more responsibilities for instructors: maintaining a regular class, studio, or community as a 'safe space'; developing an intuition about when to push a student to go deeper and when to give a student space; knowing when to advise a student to get outside help; and also taking care of themselves as they take on a challenging role in students' development. Many instructors intuitively take on this role, giving short 'dharma talks' about the meaning of poses or the meaning of one's approach, employing gentle touch to not only 'correct' a pose but also help calm an upset student, encouraging emotionally sensitive awareness and relaxation of long-held muscular tension.

By recognizing both the psychological value and risks involved in yoga practice, those of us in the yoga community have the opportunity to grow the field and increase its ability to serve students. Many yoga practitioners have long denounced the public assumption that yoga is merely 'stretching,' so we can work in tandem with psychotherapists and researchers to share the value of our knowledge.

A student's response to a teacher can bring up psychodynamics similar to that of a therapist–client relationship. Transference, the redirection of feelings from an old relationship onto a new one, is always possible, and the challenging nature of some postures can activate this. Effective teachers have a number of styles ranging from demanding (more effort, deeper stretches, 'Get that leg up there!') to supportive, allowing a wide variety of expressions of the taught *asana*. While no style can be considered 'correct,' everyone has experiences with all kinds of approaches in both schooling and personal lives, and some of those experiences can carry emotional charge. Transference can be a long-term experience over many classes with the same teacher, or just a momentary trigger in a new class. The student may not even be aware of why he or she suddenly feels a different way. This is not necessarily a bad thing, but viewing what goes on in a yoga class as something that parallels what goes on in a therapy session can allow both sides to handle any transference issues with sensitivity and patience.

Possibilities for Therapy

Psychotherapists with an interest in and knowledge of yoga have a great opportunity to deepen their work with their clients. By monitoring the client's inner dialogue while in class, the pair can glean more general information about the client's responses to challenge, limitation, and even achievement. If a therapist is well-versed in yoga, he or she can ask a client to repeatedly work with a particular *asana* that represents an aspect of being they might be working on developing, either in a session or throughout the week, and pay attention to the thoughts and feelings that arise when he or she takes on that bodily shape. On a less involved level, therapists can suggest yoga as a form of physical exercise or stress reduction. Symbolically, the act of showing up for a yoga practice can teach self-discipline and self-care, and carries its own sensory and emotional rewards to reinforce the effort. Mental health workers can even take continuing education classes that certify them to use simple yoga techniques such as breath work and body awareness with clients.

This does not just happen on an individual level, but can be a community-wide change. When community centers, prisons, and religious groups begin offering yoga to their communities, the greater psychological health can be part of a large-scale intervention. As parents learn to take care of themselves and manage their own energetic and emotional states, they can be more responsive to their children's spoken and unspoken needs. As students learn to focus in school, they perform better and learn more. As multiple members of a community become better able to care for themselves, they become better able to care for other members of the community as well. Yoga's effectiveness as a regulatory technique for excitation can help to reduce violence and aggression when it is part of community programming.

Maintaining physical health and learning to manage stress and uncomfortable emotions are, of course, habits universally necessary for people who are healthy, at risk, or suffering from a mental illness. This may seem like common sense, but our medical system is designed on a pathology-cure model, meaning that action is not taken until uncomfortable symptoms or at least clear risk factors for disease emerge. When a disease does emerge, it is treated as a distinct part of the person. When one studies anatomy and energy through yoga practice, however, the old song about the hip bone being connected to the leg bone rings true – a misalignment or poorly healed injury in one part of the whole person can easily manifest elsewhere. 'Babying' a broken toe can lead to stress injuries in the knee or hip, and a difficult conversation can show up later as tight, hunched shoulders. Developing a daily practice that strengthens and energizes all of the bodily and energetic systems in this way prevents widespread injury and illness. As a complementary therapy for depression, for example, yoga develops physical energy that allows a person to build physical strength to create a subtle sense of empowerment, and a general sense of acceptance, well-being, and compassion toward self and others.

Through approaching one another's emotional well-being with an understanding of how it thrives and is afflicted both in mystical and scientific terms; by considering the inner dialogue and relationship between thoughts, feelings, and body that occurs on the mat; and by strengthening our approach, we can begin to use yoga as a tool for a whole-person approach to health. What is happening while one is learning yoga is more than just recovery or resiliency. It is a path of personal growth toward self-actualization. By integrating yoga into our strategies for getting and staying healthy, we can redefine the way we think of health – perhaps as an ever-increasing capacity to do whatever we want or need to do in life, and to enjoy it along the way.

ABBY THOMPSON

CHAPTER 14

THE PATH TO HAPPINESS BEGINS
WITH A JOURNEY INSIDE

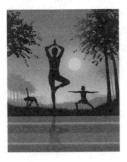

A long-awaited break from the rain allowed for a mid-afternoon walk and some fresh air – nothing like some quality time with Mother Nature to get the blood circulating after being cooped up and tortured by chalk dust all day. Puddles were still fresh from a soaking rain and, being in a 'Mon daze,' I didn't notice the puddle just in front of me. Just as I was about to step right in, a voice in my head gently advised me to 'step around puddle, Jimmy; step in and get wet foot.' This may not read quite like Yoda – the 800-year-old Jedi knight – but all I could think of was his voice as I stepped around the puddle. Next thing you know I was walking to the beat of the wisdoms of Yoda before realizing that I should be thinking about *yoga* and philosophy, not *Yoda* and philosophy. Although different topics, there are some similarities.

Experience helped to make Yoda wise – I guess when you live to be over 800 years old you experience a thing or two in your life. Yoda was able to look below the surface, understanding that the root of evil and destruction lie within a person, and the *force*, our inner strength and spirit, can conquer evil. To look into one's self is to discover who one is. Now, I am not professing to be Yoda or a Jedi knight; since I am a 'newbie'

Yoga – Philosophy for Everyone: Bending Mind and Body, First Edition.
Edited by Liz Stillwaggon Swan.
© 2012 John Wiley & Sons, Inc. Published 2012 by John Wiley & Sons, Inc.

to yoga, I am not ready to 'philosophize' or be a salesman for one particular style of yoga. What I can speak to is my own personal story with yoga – a first-hand account of my discovery of yoga and the effect it has had on my life.

Since I began practicing yoga a few months ago, I have experienced a deeper recognition of myself and the world around me – a feeling of clarity. The more I practice, the more I feel a sense of my mind and body purging themselves of the trash of negative thoughts. I did not realize what a taxing effect this battle between my body and mind had taken on me. Having tried other avenues to happiness and just ended up more miserable, I have discovered that yoga provides a path of sustained happiness through sustained awareness.

As you read this essay, I hope you can sense my enthusiasm and passion for yoga. I do not make a grandiose infomercial guarantee that yoga is another 'end all be all' quick fix to anxiety, depression, and anger. Those claims would be disrespectful to those who have spent their lives studying and practicing yoga. We are all created differently and, although we may drink from the same cup, only one of us may get drunk. Therefore, it is important to realize that my experiences may not be the same as those of others who practice yoga.

The Emotional and Physical Toll of Anxiety

I guess the best time to begin this journey is the night of December 18, 2009 (I could take you all the way back but that would ruin my big memoir plans). I was sprawled out on my couch, tucked away from the cruel world that waited outside my door. I was feeling relieved to have made it through another day in one piece, though my body felt like it had gone through a twelve-round fight with Mike Tyson in his prime. Each day had become nothing more than a repetitive bore – man, could I empathize with Bill Murray's character in *Groundhog Day*, living a life of purgatory punishment – the dreaded 'same old same old.' Each morning began with the curse of the alarm clock. Do I really have to get up and do this again? Why can't I just stay under the covers?' By seven am, I had already punished myself with more negative thoughts and emotions than most people experience in a month, fearing what the day may bring. Are the kids going to listen to me today? Am I a good teacher? Do I have enough money in my savings account? What are others saying about me? These questions were followed by intense anxiety, the kind that grips your insides, grinding them into a gnawing sensation that rips apart the insides.

When shaving, I saw a face that was worn from perpetual worry and sadness. My make-up – a toothy smile and a face of happiness – masked how I really felt. I looked ten years older than I was. My body was bloated and out of shape, I was physically and emotionally exhausted, and when I felt motivated to exercise I could not muster the strength to get out the door. The antidepressants I was taking were just numbing my problems. I knew I was upset or anxious about something, but I could not reach down to find the cause. Attempts to self-medicate made me lethargic, sleepy, and unmotivated. Most afternoons were passed away in a stupor of sleep, too exhausted to move. I knew I had to get a hold of my life, but I continued to make excuses for who and what I had become. Excuses blocked the true source of my pain. It is difficult to accept responsibility, but that is where true change begins.

'Once in a while you get shown the light in the strangest of places if you look at it right.'

Scarlet Begonias, lyrics by Robert Hunter

Strange things happen when we least expect it. On this particular December, I got the motivation to get off the couch and do something I had not done in quite some time: stretch. In a trance-like state, I felt that weird feeling you get when you stand up too quickly. I made my way over to my fireplace, knelt down in what I later learned was the *kapalbhati* position (kneeling), and felt what can best be described as excruciating pleasure. It had been years since I had last stretched and my body was paying me back for years of neglect. The muscles and tendons in my thighs and hamstrings were wound up like rubber-band balls (you could say I was 'tightly wound') and felt like they would snap at any moment. Despite the pain, I didn't want to quit the stretch; I actually enjoyed the sensation of pain and the pleasure that came with it. I could feel the flow of fresh blood cooling the areas that hurt the most. It was like instant hydration for my body: muscles, ligaments, and tendons being nourished by the flow of oxygenated blood.

Though my first yoga experience lasted less than a minute, my body was basking in the enjoyment of released tension. Standing up, the cool sensation of tingling blood remained. I felt rejuvenated. I made my way over to my chair, sank deep into the cushions, and inhaled the deepest, belly-expanding breath. As I inhaled, my stomach inflated like a balloon (a big balloon for that matter). For ten minutes I sat and watched my stomach expand and deflate with each exhale. The knots in my stomach were slowly coming undone. My concentration was solely on my breath, ignoring the usual brain noise typically intruding into my waking thoughts. For once, I was not thinking about money, relationships, work, family, or any of my other stresses and anxieties; my only focus was my breath and the relaxing sensation taking over my body. This may sound so simple, *to stretch and breathe*, but for someone who had couldn't take a minute to slow his thinking down – unable to get hold of the racing mind – it was a huge step forward. Little did I know it, but on this night in December I introduced myself to the world of yoga. Though my routine was far from perfect (hell, I didn't even know I was doing yoga), it was the foundation for more research and practice. I wish I had filmed myself in those early poses just to see how tight my body and mind were. It would have been very interesting to see my progress over the course of time.

Decluttering the Body and Mind

As yoga became a daily practice, I noticed feelings coming to the surface. Some nights I would experience intense happiness while others I would feel paralyzing, deep-rooted emotions of fear and anxiety. Over the course of my lifetime, I had allowed self-defeating emotions to create my own anxiety and misery. Fear of failure, fear of death, fear of being alone, fear of what others thought about me – whether in terms of my personality, the way I dressed, or the length of my hair. It would not take a psychologist to tell you that fear was the source of my problems, blocking much of my energy flow. Whereas I used to run from feelings such as these, or attempt to bury and 'drown' them away, with yoga there was nowhere to run. I could allow the negative emotions to ruin my yoga session or I could choose to let go of all the negative feelings. My journal entry from one particular night in January, after less than one month of practicing yoga, captures my experience of confronting fear.

January 8, 2010: 'The Color of Anxiety' A peaceful feeling of deep relaxation passes over me. My mind is free, the blood flows gently through my body, hydrating areas of pain. Muscles are relaxing, and I can feel the knots of tension slowly coming undone. My eyelids project a bright sunshine-filled sky, I am calm and at peace, basking in the radiance of the sun. All of a sudden, without any warning, like a summer storm coming off the ocean, my peaceful tranquility turned to darkness. Panic and worry set in, I am lifted from my body in this strange three-dimensional, out of body experience. I feel lost and confused, realizing that I have been here before. I am on top of a building, looking up at a dark and evil sky. As a kid I would have this same nightmare whenever I had a fever, the feeling of falling from a building, and awaking just before I hit the ground. Tonight, I refuse to allow myself to worry as I have done so many times in the past. I will not let my fear get the best of me. I can control my thoughts, and I refuse to leave my peaceful state. I take a few deep belly breaths and feel a sense of calmness return to my heart and mind. My body relaxes and once again I feel focused on the moment in front of me. A gray sky fades into a bright orange and yellow; I have weathered a storm.

My fear of heights stemmed from a fear of falling and losing control. Therefore, I needed to do whatever I could to control the situation. This had become my channel of thinking for quite some time, and it seemed to only be progressing. Eventually, something has to give; if fear is not dealt with, it only builds up. Think of it like this: if we never take the time to bring out the garbage, it just piles up, becoming smellier and filthier. Our homes become cluttered with trash. Garbage does not magically go away; we have to throw it out ourselves. The mind and body behave in a similar way; they become receptacles for our negative thoughts. We can hide from the source of our pain, but it is not going to go away; like trash, it just builds over time, rotting the body and mind from the inside out. Yoga has helped me to break through the layers of defense, allowing for positive flow of energy, channeling through the body and mind, clearing away the toxic buildup of stress.

Finding the source of the problem may require working through piles of trash, and, believe me, it stinks! My decluttering was at times awful: nights in tears and frustration at the recognition of pain I had caused myself and those around me. Coming to grips and making peace with my past was not easy, but it was a necessary step for my progress. In order to 'let go' I had to know what it was that I was letting go of. Through yoga I have become more adept at such recognition; therefore, when I do experience a feeling of stress, or fear, I am able to calm myself through breath and focus, balancing the mind and body.

Slowing Down the Breath, Slowing Down the Mind

My problems are no worse than problems you have experienced. In fact, I am willing to bet there are many out there who would gladly exchange their problems for mine. I have three good friends who have passed away and who would have taken my problems on in a heartbeat in exchange for just one more day to be alive. I was my own worst enemy, taking small, tangible issues and throwing gasoline on them, igniting them into a raging inferno. I diagnosed myself as a 'mental cutter,' one who takes a small problem and immediately thinks of all the worst-case scenarios. Someone who 'cuts' usually does it to cover up a deeper pain or fear, or as a call for help. The mental cutter cuts himself through painful thinking in an attempt to mask deeper fears or pain.

Here is an example. Let's say my girlfriend wants to stay at her place for the night, using the time to catch up on her own life. Immediately I would think that something must be wrong with me. I must have done something to make her not want to see me; I must be the issue. I would then begin a barrage of negative thinking: 'Why does she not want to do anything with me tonight? Is she sick of me? Bored? Does she not care about me? We are going to break up, I just know it!' My reaction to many situations was an 'end of the world' mentality, feeling that every situation I thought about was predetermined to have a bad ending.

Yoga helps me to slow down my thinking in stressful situations, allowing me to focus on the situation and the origin of my thinking, as opposed to reacting at first thought. In writing this essay, I went back to a journal entry from March of 2010:

> I am my own worst enemy. I am impulsive; when I feel threatened I lash out in defense. I want to strike first before I get struck, must be my old football mentality coming out. I always feel like I am protecting myself, like I have to be on guard for all the worst possible situations. I tend to react before thinking, and thus, the reason my reactions get me into embarrassing and regrettable situations.

As I reflected on the entry, I wrote down the word 'accountability' and circled it, and then wrote the following: 'you did not create this situation, but you sure as hell can control your own response.' Yoga is about slowing down the mind and body, focusing on the feeling of energy rising up through the core of the body and on up to the top of the head. If one is consumed by one's own selfish thoughts (and that is what I was, a selfish thinker) then yoga loses its proper meaning.

When most people think of yoga, myself included, they think of someone twisted in some pretzel-like posture; but, as I have found, breath in yoga is just as important as any posture. In fact, as I have come to learn, improper breathing leads to improper posture, and, hence, the yoga session is for naught. An impulsive person reacts spontaneously; they do not think about the situation, they simply react based on the first thoughts that come to mind. Impulsive breathing, or shallow breathing, is short and rapid, and the resulting lack of oxygen leads to feeling in a state of hyperventilation. So, even when I was not 'stressed,' my body and mind were in a state of preparation for a stressor to arise, and therefore I never felt calm or relaxed.

When in yoga stretch, I do not allow my mind to focus on the stress of pain; instead I channel my focus onto my breath, concentrating on the deep rhythmic inhale and exhale. I feel my body and mind begin to slow, and eventually to calm. What I do in yoga is only important if it is also being applied outside of practice; otherwise I am no different from a great practice player who cannot play at the same level in the big game. I created what I call my 'five-second rule.' When faced with a stressful situation, I take a deep breath, inhaling for five seconds, holding for two, and exhaling until my belly is deflated. After, I ask myself the following questions (in my head, of course, unless I am alone): Is it worth it to get upset? Will I make the problem worse if I get upset? Sometimes, a deep breath is not enough, and I need to distract myself or clear my mind even before breathing. At times like these, a long walk, or journal venting, or a conversation with a trusted friend can do wonders.

Learning to Live Free of Fear

If you had asked me a year ago how my life was, you probably would have been greeted with a big, wide smile. I would have said how great my life was, my smile masking what lay beneath the surface. That is why those reading this who know me may be surprised by what you have read. You see, by nature I am stubborn and do not want people to feel sorry for me or try to help me. I did not want to admit I had a problem, so I continued on, piling one problem onto the next. My anger was nothing more than a mask, covering up my fears. A year ago my life had become consumed by my fear, negatively affecting my job, relationships, friendships, and living habits. If there was a rock bottom, I had arrived – and if I wasn't there yet I sure as hell didn't want to discover it.

Although I did not set out to find yoga, I am fortunate for my accidental discovery. Yoga has changed my life, but yoga by itself did not change me. Yoga, like Yoda for that matter, has been more of a teacher and a guiding voice of reason – not dictating to me as much as coaching me, helping me to recognize what lies within, and helping me to gain confidence in myself as a person. Yoga is not a pill you pop when you want to 'feel better.' It is a process that takes time to develop. It is a marathon, more than a sprint, and I know in today's quick-fix world something that takes time is sometimes considered not an option. But hey, as I said, yoga may not be for everyone.

Yoga, a Gateway Drug?

So, what began as a one-night accident continues to expand my body and mind every day. Each morning begins with a cup of joe and twenty minutes of light stretching ('morning worship,' as I call it) and some mindful meditation. I look forward to my nightly routine of a full hour of yoga as a therapeutic end to the day, a chance to deflate and let go of all the left-over emotions. For me, there was an instant connection between yoga and the positive interaction I was experiencing emotionally and physically; the mind and body working together as one cohesive unit, coexisting in balance rather than battling for turf supremacy. I began to identify areas of my body where I held the most pain. The hamstrings and lower back held fear, my stomach held anxiety and fear, and my shoulders and upper body held insecurities. It is very enlightening to discover that the body is like a road map for the mind. I feel like yoga has taught me more than any course I took as student in college or graduate school. What is especially cool is that I am my own professor! Everything I have learned and continue to learn comes from my own experiences and from my own body and mind. I am my own guru.

We all have experiences to learn from, it's just that many of us become trapped by our own thoughts and are therefore blinded by the surface and unable to look deep inside for the source of our problems. Though I could not put my finger on it immediately, I was aware of a sense of transformation and change within my body and mind. On the surface, the effects of yoga are visible – my body is more toned and I feel ten years younger. My physical and emotional flexibility are at levels I have never before experienced, and I feel more 'in the flow' of my life. Life is not perfect, and neither am I. There are still plenty of bad days, and moments that test my 'yogic resolve.' I still am prone to periods of gloominess, but I recognize my behaviors and work to let go of the feelings causing them. Someday it may come naturally, but at this point in my life I am just happy to be happy. I have learned a lot about myself over the last twelve months. Playing the role of my own therapist, I have been able to gain great insight into myself. Yoga has done more for me than stretch and tone my body; it has helped me to open doors of perception that had always been there, just not yet opened. Yoga did not actually open the doors; I had to do that myself, which is why I have felt my self-confidence grow so much. I am proud of what I have accomplished through my own hard work.

Maybe I should have learned yoga from a master, or taken a class before diving into it. But, for someone who has always been a better 'self-taught' student, I am glad I chose not to. I did not have the self-confidence to sit in a room with others out of fear of being judged. I am happy to feel that 'of the true reflection inside the mirror speaks; hide from what we try to conceal, we cannot,' as Yoda would say.

PART 4

YAMAS AND *NIYAMAS*:
ETHICS AND YOGA

CHAPTER 15

GET OUT OF MY WAY! I'M LATE FOR YOGA!

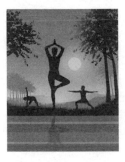

Once upon a time, there lived an evil king named Daksha who was not at all happy with his son-in-law Shiva, the most powerful of all yogic deities. Daksha was having a huge ceremonial sacrifice in his kingdom and refused to invite Shiva. When Daksha's daughter, Sati, became aware that her husband was shunned she became terribly upset and showed up alone at the ceremony, where she threw herself on the sacrificial fire in protest against her father's behavior. When Shiva found out about his wife's death he became very angry, and tore a lock from his hair and threw it to the Earth. Out of this fury Virabhadra, a ferocious and ruthless warlord, was born. Shiva instructed Virabhadra to destroy Daksha's kingdom in revenge for Sati's death. Virabhadra did just that.

This is the story behind the yoga *asana* (posture) known as *virabhadrasana*: warrior pose. In warrior I pose, the practitioner stands with his or her legs far apart front to back and, keeping the back leg fully extended, bends the front leg into a right-angle with the arms extended overhead.

This posture was meant to be performed in the spirit of its mythology. And what is mythology but philosophy put into story form? The

Yoga – Philosophy for Everyone: Bending Mind and Body, First Edition.
Edited by Liz Stillwaggon Swan.
© 2012 John Wiley & Sons, Inc. Published 2012 by John Wiley & Sons, Inc.

practitioner of this pose is to feel empowered enough to destroy, not beastly people like Daksha, as in the story, but rather his or her own beastly nature.

At another time long ago there lived Rama, a prince beloved by his people and married to Sita, who was stolen from him by his arch-rival Ravana. Rama called on the Lord of the Wind, Hanuman, to help him find Sita. Hanuman is said to have taken one incredible leap from India to a distant island where he heard Sita was being held captive. Once Sita's location was confirmed, Rama's army built a bridge to the island and, with the help of Hanuman, Sita and Rama were eventually reunited.

Hanuman's leap has been immortalized in a yoga posture known as *hanumanasana*, wherein the practitioner extends one leg forward and the other leg backward until the pelvis sits on the floor in a split-like position. The palms are to be folded in front of the heart center in honor of this deity and the loyalty and courage he stands for. Furthermore, as Lord of the Wind, Hanuman is also Lord of *pranayama*, which is the yogic art of breath control. When *pranayama* is mastered, the practitioner experiences a blissful union of his or her feminine and masculine energies that is symbolized in this legend about Sita and Rama.

But now, in this age of consumerism and commercialism in the West, these rich yoga legends and the philosophy they embody are becoming lost. The whole subject of yoga is rapidly being reduced to just another highly packaged and strongly marketed fitness technique that happens to include stretching and relaxation.

I feel it is important, therefore, that today's yoga teachers include this vast, enriching philosophy of yoga when they teach its physical practices of *asana* and *pranayama*. A reading of any of the ancient yoga texts will reveal the truth that yoga philosophy has always been integral to and inseparable from yoga practice. In fact, the true yogi was expected to incorporate his or her study of philosophy in *all* daily actions, not just 'on the mat' (which were made of deer skin back then). Addressing this point more recently, yoga master B. K. S. Iyengar, author of *Light on Yoga*, the most-referred-to yoga book on the planet today, warns that the practice of the *asanas* (postures) without the benefit of yoga philosophy is mere acrobatics. He goes on to say that a coordinated effort of all the components of yoga is required for one to win the prize of inner peace.

Furthermore, the eight basic components that comprise the whole subject of yoga are so interrelated that they are referred to as 'limbs,' thus implying that they are inseparable just as the branches of a tree stem from the same trunk. These components are: (1) rules of conduct for living in society, (2) observances of certain behavioral standards that keep one in tune with oneself, (3) the practice of yoga postures, (4) the practice of yoga breathing, (5) sensory withdrawal, (6) concentration, (7) meditation, and (8) self-realization, which is actually a result rather than a practice.

I once inherited a student who had been practicing yoga poses for a number of years without the benefit of yoga philosophy study. Running late to class one day, this student hastily tried to park her car only to smash the fender of an unoccupied parked vehicle. She eventually pulled into a spot and, ignoring what had just happened, ran into my classroom, put down her mat, and joined in. Of course I had no knowledge of what had transpired, but I did notice that her breathing was off and her poses were a little shaky. About half way through the class a police officer entered the room looking for someone who fit the description he had been given by a few unexpected eye-witnesses to this parking debacle. He soon identified my poor student and escorted her out as she cried. Had she been taught one of the basic premises of yoga philosophy, this unfortunate student would have known that disturbing the world causes it to disturb you back. Had she studied Patañjali's *Yoga Sutras*, an important contribution to the philosophy of yoga written between 100 BCE and 500 CE, she would have learned about the ten behavioral precepts that create a life free from disturbance and therefore suitable for fostering a fruitful yoga practice.

A basic principle of yoga is to act selflessly and in the best interest of others. I witnessed something interesting in this regard as I was walking to a local coffee shop. I recognized a 'yoga practitioner' friend of mine coming toward the same shop but a little further from the door than me. I waved but for some reason he didn't see me, and he put his walk in high gear and snatched the door handle right in front of me in kind of a blocking maneuver so he could get in line ahead of me. Standing behind him in the shop, I said 'hello' and he turned embarrassedly around saying he was sorry and didn't realize that it was *me* he had cut ahead of. In other words, I think he was saying that his behavior would have been okay had it not been done to a friend. What an interesting interpretation of selfless action...

No doubt, then, the philosophy of yoga should be taught so we don't all go around being 'yoga acrobats' and not caring about others. But the average student may not be at all interested in the philosophy of yoga. For example, how could I convince a young mother with three kids that multi-tasking is inconsistent with yoga philosophy? Or a sports fan that competition is considered 'non-yogic'? If I were to push the issue, I would surely lose these students and probably turn them off to yoga, which would be a shame. Many teachers fear philosophy can be too 'heady,' vague, or subject to opinion and therefore shy away from teaching it. They therefore emphasize the more tangible and sellable yoga 'products' known as *asana* (postural exercises) and *pranayama* (breath work) so they can keep their classes well attended and pay the studio rent. And understandably so.

One morning I decided to begin one of my classes with a short tribute to Patañjali, the sage mentioned above and author of the first systematized treatise on yoga. There is a well-known invocation to him that I started to read to the class, being careful not to chant it as is traditionally done. After about the third or fourth sentence one of my newer students stood up, stated his objection that this was, 'all very uncomfortable for him,' and walked out, demanding a full refund for the cost of his ten-class card.

Another time I was talking about the yogic precepts of contentment and non-hoarding in class. Afterwards a rather avid student who was working hard to improve his position in the stock firm he worked for came up to talk with me. 'You mean if I keep practicing yoga I'll lose my competitive edge, my need to think big and save money for trust funds for my kids?' he questioned. 'Well, in way, *yes*,' I said. I never saw him again.

So, what is a teacher to do? When I was in college I read a study that was conducted concerning child behavior. A whole bunch of kids were confined to a large room where they were observed by a team of psychologists every day for something like two months. In this room were all sorts of toys, games, and other things the kids loved to play with. Food was also made available for the choosing. There was candy, ice cream, pop corn, soda, and the like, but also vegetables, chicken, fish, potatoes, and so on. Guess what? After a few weeks of 'sweets binging,' the kids began to choose a healthy, balanced diet all on their own.

Assuming we could project the findings of this study on adult behavior to a certain degree, it could be an effective way to bring yoga philosophy into yoga classes. In other words, yoga teachers might consider simply providing it, but not preaching it, and the students may eventually come to 'taste' it!

I have found that a good way to provide yoga philosophy is to give *asana* and *pranayama* instructions with subliminal philosophical messages embedded in them. Instead of just saying 'stretch your legs,' I may instruct my students to 'extend your legs so they are straight and true,' thereby offering the yogic precept of 'truth' in a non-preachy way. In *pranayama* I may say, 'make your exhalations as an offering and receive your inhalations as a blessing so your practice has a sense of reverence.' In this way, the richness of yoga philosophy is experienced in a useful way by the students and it takes on a real value to them.

Regarding the readiness of a student to receive yoga philosophy, I once heard a wise teacher say, 'you can't pull a flower out from its bud; it will blossom when it is ready and not before.' (Obviously this teacher never heard of forced blooming, but that's not the point.) So, by offering these subliminal philosophy messages as part of my practical teaching, I'm really not making anyone uncomfortable, and, for the student who is ready, the message will be heard.

For example, after a particular class in which I was teaching some rigorous standing poses and making statements such as 'stand on your own two feet' and 'stand for truth,' one of my students came up to me a little teary-eyed and said, as she was pulling off her engagement ring, 'thank you; you made me realize that John is not the man for me.' She realized that, in truth, she was in the relationship simply because she feared living alone.

In summary then, yes, yoga philosophy should be introduced to the students of yoga today; however, truly 'knowing' yoga philosophy is very different than knowing 'about' yoga philosophy. Recall that 'even the devil can quote the scriptures....' To know truth, then, one has to live in truth. This is the real purpose of the practice of yoga poses and breath work – to provide a practical, real experience wherein one can explore the tenets of the philosophy of this noble subject. A good yoga teacher weaves this knowledge into the physical instructions given to the class. A back-bending pose, therefore, is not just a 'backbend,' but an expansion from the innermost self to the outer reaches of consciousness, and an opening of the heart to heaven.

CHAPTER 16

YOGA OFF THE MAT

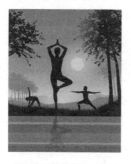

How should the Yoga Practitioner Live?

No matter who you are, simply practicing yoga does not make you a better, more moral person. We all know yogis or yoginis – including ourselves – who are at times egotistical, vain, impatient, and competitive, even in the yoga classroom. And, fifteen minutes after class, it's back to road rage, negative energy, addictions, and judgmental attitudes. It is easy to become one with the universe on the mat, but hard to do so off it.

So how should yoga practitioners live and connect their experience of yoga on the mat with their lives off it? I began practicing yoga in earnest a decade ago in New Orleans, and fellow practitioners, as you might guess, were nightclub musicians, graduate students, waitresses, and bartenders who drank, smoked, ate fried shrimp 'po-boys,' and partied during Mardi Gras. Their lifestyles – like mine – were virtuous in the eyes of other New Orleanians, but seemed incompatible with what yoga gurus espoused as the good yogic life.

Yoga – Philosophy for Everyone: Bending Mind and Body, First Edition.
Edited by Liz Stillwaggon Swan.
© 2012 John Wiley & Sons, Inc. Published 2012 by John Wiley & Sons, Inc.

Just as the physical practice of yoga can accommodate a wide variety of personalities, aptitudes, and abilities, so can yogic ethics or morality. A single ideal of a virtuous yogi or yogini simply does not exist. People's actions must be understood in the context of their community, their culture, and their way of life, as well as in recognition that each of us is on an individual journey of growth and development. What is virtuous for a yogi in New Orleans will be different from what is virtuous for a yogi in Mysore, Paris, or San Francisco. Although this may sound very Zen and hip, it doesn't mean that 'anything goes.'

In order to help yoga practitioners have a better idea of what it means to live in a yogic way, this essay will outline the virtues and morals that it is especially important for yoga practitioners to take from their practice on the mat into their lives off the mat. The term I will use to describe the virtues that are uniquely espoused by the yoga community is 'yogic virtue.' The idea of yogic virtue I develop here is rooted in the yoga practice itself and its current social context. Although yogic ethical teachings (such as those outlined in classic yogic texts such as Patañjali's second century BCE *Yoga Sutras* or Hindu scriptures such as the *Bhagavad Gita*) are important, they need to be understood within a wider context of ethical action. The best theoretical construct available for interpreting such texts is 'virtue ethics' (using the terminology of contemporary moral philosophy). A virtue ethic advocates individual development of certain virtues, rather than following strict moral rules. Much like yoga, the development of these virtues requires repetition and practice. Yoga ethics is only *one kind* of virtue ethic, and the idea of yogic virtue that I will develop here aims primarily to be of use to Western yoga practitioners in the twenty-first century.

Yoga Ethics: More than *Yamas* and *Niyamas*

In order to flesh out the idea of 'yogic virtue,' I will explore the virtues that are rooted in the *asanas*, or the physical practice of yoga. This is because a yoga practice itself can give guidance regarding moral virtue. Taking to heart even the simplest yoga concepts, such as 'open your heart,' 'relax and breathe deeply,' and 'focus and calm your mind,' can be transformative in the physical yoga practice as well as in one's life off the mat. Moreover, people bring much of what they need to grow morally with them to the yoga practice. All yoga practitioners have received years of moral instruction independently of yoga: 'do not lie, cheat, or steal,' 'respect others,' 'tell the truth,' 'have integrity,' 'be kind, generous, and compassionate,' 'develop your talents.' These moral injunctions are ubiquitous in most cultures and are consistent with the teachings in the *Yoga Sutras*, not to mention the Ten Commandments and the Buddhist Noble Eightfold Path. Those who practice yoga (as we understand it today) can develop the yogic virtues that are relevant to life off the yoga mat by reflecting on and implementing into their daily lives the lessons they learn about yoga on the mat.

Does this mean we need not study classical yogic teachings to learn how to be better yogis and yoginis? We should, but even these classical yogic texts must be interpreted and placed in the wider context of ethical action. That is what I aim to do here by demonstrating how the broad moral framework of 'virtue ethics' can be used to interpret yogic ethical teachings. This approach emphasizes the *process* of seeking yogic virtue rather than the *product* of a vice-free life.

Consider Patañjali's *Yoga Sutras*. This text is the theoretical source of all the schools of yoga, and revered teachers such as B. K. S. Iyengar and K. Pattabhi Jois used it as the basis of their writings on yoga practice. Thus, it is useful to know its teachings in order to understand why yogic ethics should be understood as a kind of virtue ethic. Patañjali outlines eight limbs (or dimensions) of yoga. The *yamas* and *niyamas* are the first two of Patañjali's eight limbs of yoga, and *asana* (or the physical practice of yoga) is the third. The *yamas* include the five 'restraints' of non-violence, truthfulness, non-stealing, moderation or non-excess, and non-hoarding; and the *niyamas* are the 'observances' of purity, contentment, austerity or self-discipline, self-study, and devotion to a higher power. What precisely do the *yamas* and *niyamas* require? Many authors and gurus have discussed them at length, and these discussions can be found easily by an interested student. But, instead of explicating the nuances of these concepts and applying them to modern life, I offer a context for understanding these teachings more generally, to see how we can use them in life off the yoga mat.

Yogic ethical teachings such as the *yamas* and *niyamas* may plausibly be interpreted as recommending that people develop certain *virtues* rather than recommending that people follow strict moral *principles*. The text lends itself to this kind of interpretation, given that it does not say anything specific about contemporary moral concerns such as, for example, eating meat, drinking alcohol or caffeine, or giving to charity. There is, of course, a long history of Hindu commentaries on the *Sutras*

❡ JULINNA OXLEY

(and the *Gita*) that do recommend performing or avoiding such actions. Even contemporary yoga teachers interpret these concepts as traditional moral principles. For example, Jivamukti yoga founder Sharon Gannon asserts that the five *yamas* of restraint – especially *ahimsa* or non-violence – support a vegetarian diet.[1] If one were to interpret the yogic teachings on non-violence, truthfulness, non-stealing, moderation, and non-hoarding as moral *principles*, then I agree that they recommend that yoga practitioners be sensitive to the way that we treat animals and, therefore, not eat meat.

But this approach to interpreting the text tends to emphasize performing outward actions rather than cultivating an inward, rational understanding of the virtues. In fact, emphasizing that the *yamas* and *niyamas* require particular *actions* over and against the development of particular *character traits* seems to go against the message of the *Yoga Sutras* and the practice of yoga more generally. This is not to say that the way that we treat animals is unimportant; indeed, this issue deserves considerable moral reflection and an investigation of contemporary farming practices. But, because yogic teachings are supposed to speak to individual practitioners, are supposed to be a guide to the practice, and are supposed to be wrestled with by each person on his or her own unique journey, it seems somewhat counterintuitive for these teachings to be used to recommend a particular action or way of life for all yogis and yoginis. It may be better to understand yogic teachings, such as the *yamas* of restraint and the *niyamas* of observances, as recommending moral virtues, or personal qualities and characteristics that need to be developed, rather than as moral commands that require particular actions or a particular lifestyle. As B. K. S. Iyengar writes in his commentary on Patañjali's idea of *ahimsa*, 'merely because a man is a vegetarian, it does not follow that he is non-violent by temperament or that he is a yogi ... Blood-thirsty tyrants may be vegetarians, but violence is a state of mind, not a diet.'[2]

Iyengar's point regarding temperament captures the distinction I am making between an approach to ethics that emphasizes the development of moral virtue and one that emphasizes the performance of particular actions. Yogic ethics are best understood as a kind of virtue ethic because – in the same way that yoga practice is modified to suit each individual's life context, personal aptitude, ability, and interest – moral growth and the development of virtue are also relative to the individual. To see this, let us examine how the virtue approach to ethics conceives the moral life by articulating its core components.

The Elements of Virtue Ethics

Virtue ethics is one of three major ethical theories regarding the good life in contemporary moral philosophy (the others are utilitarianism and Kantian ethics or deontology). What follows is a summary of the main elements of virtue ethics, as it is generally understood in the Western analytic philosophy tradition. This will provide both a framework for interpreting yogic teachings and a better understanding of how ethics is related to the practice of yoga.

Character and habituation

According to virtue ethics, the good life is pursued over the course of one's life, and each person is a work in progress. Virtues must be developed, and they require repetition and practice. This means that it is not enough to perform just one generous action. In order to *become* generous, one must have the emotions and thoughts that motivate generosity, and one must have them on a regular basis. When one acquires the disposition to give to others, generosity becomes second nature. This is what it means to develop character or certain virtues: habitually fostering certain emotional responses, desires, and perceptions enables one to develop a particular kind of attitude or disposition. To develop virtue, people should identify their weaknesses, such as their tendency toward vices such as stinginess, and try to work on controlling their feelings and thoughts so as to develop virtues such as generosity. This approach does not so much recommend that people perform (or not perform) particular *actions*, but that they develop certain qualities of mind and heart.

Virtue

According to virtue ethics, people need to develop virtues instead of vices. Aristotle, who is considered the father of virtue ethics, defines a virtue as a quality or character that enables an object (or person) to perform its function well.[3] For example, a knife's greatest virtue is its sharpness. A dull knife cannot perform well the function of cutting. So, what is the function of the human being, and what enables a human being to perform its function well? Aristotle answers that the function of a human being is to use reason to make good choices, deliberate, and take care of things. One should develop virtues that help one perform this function well; otherwise, one will live badly. This is why we need virtues: they enable us to live well and flourish.

So which virtues should we develop? There is not much agreement about which are the best or most important, and the virtues one highly esteems will largely depend on one's culture, values, and community. Aristotle defines a virtue as 'the mean between two extremes,' and those extremes are both vices.[4] Now this doesn't mean that Aristotle is advocating moderation in all things. Take, for example, the virtue of courage. It is the mean between the excess of courage (foolhardiness) and the deficiency of courage (cowardice). In Aristotle's day and age, virtues such as magnanimity, courage, and justice were highly esteemed. Today, Western society reveres somewhat different ones: independence, industriousness, creativity, efficiency, and sympathy.

Practical reasoning

According to virtue ethical theory, developing virtues is not easy. One must use practical reasoning to determine which virtue to perform in any particular situation; that is, one must deliberate on how to be virtuous at the right time, in the right way, and in the right manner, without excess or deficiency. Since people are different, and find themselves in differing situations, people will be virtuous in different ways, and need not perform the exact same action in order to be considered virtuous. This is because virtues are found, as Aristotle says, in the mean 'relative to us' not 'in the object' (or in itself) because people are different.[5] People are born with different personalities, needs, abilities, and goals in life, and so the way that each person is virtuous will be unique to that person. Virtue is relative to the individual's disposition, social situation, and quest for lifetime happiness, and each person must use practical reasoning when deciding how to act in any given situation, including one's choice of yoga style, studio, or class.

Community

Importantly, virtue ethics emphasizes that the good life is lived in a community, among people who espouse and promote a particular set of virtues. The community is a crucial part of virtue ethics because it sets the boundaries on morality, so that morality is not a free-for-all. The virtues that are esteemed by any particular community really *are* the virtues its members should seek to develop. In addition, the community has a responsibility to encourage the performance of certain virtues, so that the members of that community can practice and develop those virtues with accountability.

This concludes my brief summary of the elements of virtue ethics. If we look at yoga, we find that the yogic virtues that are laid out in the *Yoga Sutras* (such as non-violence, truthfulness, moderation, non-hoarding, purity, contentment, and self-discipline) suggest a unique ideal of the virtuous person. This ideal is composed of virtues that are particularly relevant to yoga practitioners interested in connecting yoga to their everyday lives, and the core idea of yogic virtue can be summed up as an ethic of *mindfulness* – awareness of one's own self and awareness of others. Interpreting yogic teachings as a virtue ethic also requires that yogis and yoginis develop the virtues that are espoused within the yoga community. As I show momentarily, yogic teachings and the yoga community are diverse enough to recommend a wide range of virtues so that yogic virtue can be achieved in a variety of ways.

Understood as a virtue ethic, yogic ethics is not a 'one size fits all' morality. Not only would that go against the very concept of virtue (which is highly dependent on the individual, his or her community, and his or her personal life journey), but it also goes against the nature of the yoga practice, which is highly personal and tailored to the individual. Each person's *trikonasana* (triangle pose) will look different – though some touch the floor, other practitioners will touch a knee, a thigh, or a block. But the individual practices yoga in a community with defined limits (no cell phone calls, no loud talking, and no ogling other practitioners) and a common intention (focusing one's attention and breathing deeply and carefully). As I explain below, the same goes for morality. By understanding yoga texts and teachings as a virtue ethic, practitioners can develop virtues that are central to the discipline of yoga both on and off the yoga mat.

The Yogic Virtues

Now to the main question: What does virtue ethics tell us about yoga ethics and yogic virtue? To answer this we must first decide how to learn about the yogic virtues. There are two ways we could proceed. We could investigate the classic yogic texts such as the *Yoga Sutras* or the *Bhagavad*

Gita, or we could take Aristotle's approach and ask which virtue or virtues are unequivocally espoused in the community of yoga teachers and practitioners. This is the approach I will take, as the yoga community defines what is central to the practice of yoga. So, what yogic ideals are widely espoused by the yoga community as the heart of the yoga practice?

Although many virtues are frequently mentioned in the yoga community, such as being calm, caring, sensitive, focused, and selfless, there are two ideas that are at the conceptual root of the yogic life, and from which most other yogic virtues can be derived: (1) mindfulness and (2) self-discipline or self-improvement. These two ideas capture what is unique about yogic ethics (as compared to other kinds of virtue ethics, such as care ethics or Friedrich Nietzsche's ethics of self-creativity).

What is mindfulness? Mindfulness expresses yoga's unique approach to living in the world, and is thus the paramount virtue for yogic ethics. Mindfulness involves having knowledge of the social world and the circumstances in which we find ourselves. It involves being aware of oneself; one's existence and thoughts; other beings, including their thoughts, feelings, and situations; and one's relationship to others and with the world. Mindfulness is best understood as a broad, overarching virtue from which virtues such as compassion, sympathy, sensitivity, and a loving nature may be derived. There are two aspects of mindfulness: an attitudinal component, which involves one's emotions, thoughts, feelings, and temperament, and a practical component, which involves a response to others and the taking of certain kinds of actions.

Developing an attitude of mindfulness, and thus the virtue of mindfulness, involves developing emotions and dispositions toward others that involve awareness, empathy, compassion, and sympathy, both with regard to oneself and to others. It is a state of mind and heart, and includes a focused awareness of one's mind as the seat of mental activity and an attempt to control one's thoughts and emotions so as to be more aware of oneself. Mindfulness means learning to slow down, ceasing the tendency to flit from one thought to another without reflection, and recognizing the problems associated with being motivated by stress and anxiety. The aim of cultivating an attitude of mindfulness is to become more calm, thoughtful, and aware of others rather than preoccupied with one's mental life. The method by which one achieves the virtue of mindfulness generally includes meditation (guided or individual) and relaxation (in postures such as *savasana* or seated lotus).

The active component of mindfulness, or exhibiting the virtue of mindfulness outwardly, involves performing actions that exhibit one's attitude of mindfulness. This includes, for example, showing concern for others, sharing with others, being benevolent, or giving to charity. The actions of mindfulness can be encouraged through *seva*, or service, but there are many other ways that a person could exhibit mindfulness as a virtue: mentoring others, caring for friends and family, volunteering through a local church or organization, or caring for the environment by helping to change agricultural and factory farming practices. Developing the virtue of mindfulness has led many yoga practitioners to recognize how privileged they are to practice yoga (people must have time and flexibility to squeeze in a yoga class and money to attend it), and yoga outreach is rapidly growing in the Western yoga community. A number of non-profit yoga outreach organizations have been formed in recent years to share yoga with those who do not have the privilege of yoga. Seane Corn's Off the Mat, Into the World shares yoga with the poor in Africa and elsewhere, Y.O.G.A. for Youth shares yoga with inner-city Los Angeles youth, Yoga Behind Bars provides yoga instruction for the imprisoned in Seattle, and Project Air works with Rwandan women and children who are victims of sexual assault and rape. Sharing yoga with others in this way not only exhibits mindfulness *of* others, but also gives mindfulness as a gift *to* others and is an especially interesting opportunity for service in the yoga community.

The practice of yoga as it is taught in the Western yoga community suggests a second paramount yogic virtue: developing one's abilities and talents, not just on the yoga mat but as a person. To have the disposition of self-discipline means having an attitude of care for oneself, and reflecting on one's personal and moral development. Developing the virtue of self-discipline may require caring for oneself by becoming more mentally, emotionally, and physically sound. It may include learning how to eat healthier foods, spending time with more uplifting friends, and spending one's time wisely rather than mindlessly frittering it away. Developing the inward virtue of self-discipline entails cultivating one's talents and interests, finding opportunities to develop one's career path and personal relationships, and growing as a person, seeking new interests, outlets, and challenges.

What actions exhibit the virtue of self-discipline or self-improvement? Some might argue that it is necessary to live in a healthy manner by ceasing to eat meat, drink alcohol, and smoke cigarettes. While these are admirable ways of becoming more self-disciplined, are they requirements for yogic virtue? In answering this question, is important to remember that, while the yoga community broadly emphasizes self-improvement, it does not agree on what self-improvement requires. Some communities may say that it requires dietary restrictions, and others may emphasize outreach and activism as important to self-improvement. Most practitioners follow what their community does, whether the community is defined as the school of yoga one practices (e.g., Iyengar, Ashtanga, Kundalini, Bikram, Anusara) or the city, town, or locality in which one practices yoga.

Given this, yogic virtue will by definition look different to different people in different communities, and so no specific actions are required to exhibit self-discipline. Although some have argued that yoga teachers and practitioners should not drink alcohol, this fails to recognize that people in different cultures have different lifestyles and different social and gastronomic traditions. Take my fellow practitioners in New Orleans. Although some have quit smoking and stopped drinking alcohol, and some eat healthier now than they did years ago, others do not. Some simply live, eat, and drink in moderation. The point, though, is that, for many, yoga has positively impacted their lives, and they have consciously changed in order to grow in the practice. But to say that all yoga practitioners ought to not drink alcohol or be vegetarians is counterproductive, as it precludes such practitioners from pursuing yogic virtue in their own life journey. Moreover, it fails to recognize the diversity of the yoga community. What may be right for one yogi may *not* be right for another: becoming a vegetarian, ceasing to drink alcohol and coffee, or taking a personal vow of pacifism, charity, or anti-materialism is not necessarily morally *required*. Such actions may, of course, be recommended. But whether it is one's duty to perform any of these actions largely depends on each person's needs, social situation, and aspirations.

Conclusion

The above summarizes in broad fashion the idea of yogic virtue. My goal was to introduce a unique ethical ideal rooted in the practice of yoga as it is experienced by the yoga community at large, illustrating in the process that yoga is for everyone – even the most rationalistic, materialistic, overweight, tight-hamstringed, stressed-out person you can imagine. Everyone can benefit from yoga – physically, psychologically, and morally.

Some might object that my theory of yogic virtue is not strongly supported by the Hindu texts and writings that are the roots of yoga. But this is inaccurate. In the *Bhagavad Gita*, Krishna tells Arjuna that following doctrines and principles in order to receive a higher birth in the future is contrary to the better path in life, which involves doing good things because they are good, not because they pay off. Learning the higher path and understanding what is good, he says, happens through meditation and yoga, and those who gain self-knowledge through yoga should not focus on following the rules as they appear in doctrinal writings; rather, they should seek discernment to understand their personal duty.[6]

Others might complain that the theory of yogic virtue I describe here is not specific enough to adequately guide twenty-first-century yoga practitioners. Alas, this is somewhat true: virtue ethics (and yogic virtue ethics) does not articulate simple moral formulas or principles to follow in every situation. But this is not something to rue. As in the yoga practice, moral action is up to the individual; each person must use practical reasoning to discern how to live (or practice) virtuously. Neither I, nor any writings in the *Yoga Sutras*, are well suited to tell you what to do in every situation or in every moral dilemma.

Like the practice of yoga, the morality of yogic virtue does not provide set, specific answers or universal routines for everyone. In the same way that there are multiple ways to modify postures to suit the practitioner, there are multiple ways to develop yogic virtue for those who attempt it. Cultivating and achieving yogic virtue, like the practice of yoga, is a journey of growth, a lifetime commitment, and always a work in progress.

NOTES

1 Sharon Gannon, *Yoga and Vegetarianism: The Path to Greater Health and Happiness* (San Rafael, CA: Mandala Publishing, 2008).
2 B. K. S. Iyengar, *Light on Yoga* (New York: Schocken Books, 1966), p. 32.
3 Aristotle, *Nichomachean Ethics*, translated by Terence Irwin (Indianapolis, IN: Hackett Publishing Company, 1985), Book 1, Section 7, Bekker edition (1097b22–1098a20).
4 Ibid., 1106a26–b28.
5 Ibid., 1106b1–5.

6 *Bhagavad Gita*, Chapter 2. The relevant section reads: 'Yet, the right act / Is less, far less, than the right-thinking mind. ... Scorn them that follow virtue for her gifts! / The mind of pure devotion – even here – / Casts equally aside good deeds and bad, / Passing above them. Unto pure devotion / Devote thyself ... When thy firm soul / Hath shaken off those tangled oracles / Which ignorantly guide, then shall it soar / To high neglect of what's denied or said, / This way or that way, in doctrinal writ. / Troubled no longer by the priestly lore / Safe shall it live, and sure; steadfastly bent / On meditation. This is Yog – and Peace!' Thanks to Ron Green for directing me to this passage.

CHAPTER 17

BECOMING-FROG

Yoga as Environmentalism

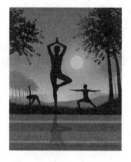 All over the world, individuals and communities are encountering the environment in unprecedented ways. Women in so-called 'developing countries' are working harder than ever to provide clean drinking water to their families; communities of color are suffering from increased cancer rates and illness due to the industrial pollution and landfills that have been placed in the very heart of their communities; and even more privileged, upper- and middle-class individuals are experiencing the impacts of polluted water and food insecurity, and the health risks that result from environmental problems. These realities and global experiences, while varied in their manifestation, are similar in the consequences they bear for all of us. Our relationship with the environment is becoming more precarious and less stable, and, as a result, life itself, both human and non-human, is degrading. Unfortunately, some will be touched by these consequences and this degradation in more severe ways than others, especially those who do not live in the shelter of the Western world. Despite the geographic differences, however, the fact remains that we, as a global community, are in need, as Vandana Shiva says, of 'Earth democracy.'

Yoga – Philosophy for Everyone: Bending Mind and Body, First Edition.
Edited by Liz Stillwaggon Swan.
© 2012 John Wiley & Sons, Inc. Published 2012 by John Wiley & Sons, Inc.

Shiva, a leading environmental activist, asserts this call for Earth democracy as a means to rethink how we should experience the environment, and as a movement toward experiencing the Earth differently. In affinity with yoga, Shiva calls for an accord between humans and the Earth. She says, 'We need a new movement, which allows us to move from the dominant and pervasive culture of violence, destruction and death to a culture of non-violence, creative peace and life.'[1] Shiva worries, like many of us concerned with the environment, not just that the way the Earth is currently treated (on both large and small scales) is destroying the very place in which we live, but also that the acts of destruction reveal a fundamental negativity in the current relationship between humans and the environment. For Shiva, the degradation of the Earth reveals a belief that humans are separate from the environment, and thus allowed to overlook our connection to the Earth. As a result, we have become arrogant inhabitants of the Earth. This is why it is critical to reconsider how we should live on Earth. Shiva's way of reconceiving how we treat, experience, and live on Earth and in the environment is the movement of Earth democracy.

I think Shiva's call for an Earth democracy is vital to how we experience tomorrow; we must consider how we can live tomorrow differently. What can I do to participate in Earth democracy? How can I realize my connection to the environment? How can I personally contribute to changing the way the Earth is treated? One of my answers to these questions is yoga. To me, yoga is one form of Earth democracy at work and, because of this, I see yoga as a political, ethical, and 'green' practice.

Many yoga practitioners have taken up the call for an environmentally conscious practice by making studios more 'green' or buying eco-friendly yoga products. But, as I see it, yoga demands that we consider nature and our environment through its very practice, both on and off the mat. From poses to breath, posture, meditation, realization, and humility, yoga is a practice of Earth democracy. And, while there are many variations of yoga practice, at the core of yoga philosophy is the affirmation of a harmonious relationship with nature, a relationship that demands yogis to connect with their surroundings. For instance, *pranayama*, the art of breathing particular to yoga, requires yogis to inhale *prana*, the vital life force of the Earth, in order to keep the body and mind healthy and focused. *Pranayama* is thus a purposive act in which yogis embody a connection to the Earth. Such purpose can be carried off the mat too. A yogi may choose to ride a bike as a means of contributing to healthy air and thus to healthy *prana*. Or, a yogi will be kind to her or his own self and to other living beings as a means to create and maintain a healthy relationship between forms of life.

Ultimately, this connection between yogis and the environment is meaningful and ethical because it demands that we be aware of ourselves, our intentions, and how we exist in the world. Because of this, yoga's conceptualization of our relationship with nature meets a pressing demand for learning how to engage with the environment anew. From my own yoga practice, I have learned and continue to learn that there is continuity between how one uses or experiences space on the yoga mat (or some other space of practice) and how one experiences the natural environment. This novel and ethical use of space that occurs because of yoga can be a means of healing the current environmental crisis.

I'm an Mammal, I'm a Reptile, I'm a Tree!

My introduction to yoga's *asanas* was the sun salutation (*surya namaskar*), a commonly practiced sequence of poses. Right now, my favorite poses are the cobra (*bhujangasana*) and the camel (*ustrasana*), and last week it was the frog pose (*bhekasana*). When I first began yoga, I enjoyed the fact that these poses open up my chest and hips while demanding flexibility in my spine. But, through practice, I came to appreciate that these poses open me up to the environment around me. Understanding how the very postures on the mat open a yogi up to the environment around her or him provides a key insight into how yoga practice is environmental.

Surya namaskar, the sun salutation, is one of the most common sequences of poses; however, ethically and philosophically, it is also one of the most significant and interesting sequences for a yogi. More specifically, saluting the sun is a means for the yogi to open herself to light, which is a means to effect self-awareness. The philosophy of yoga affirms that light is a symbol of consciousness and existence such that, without light, we would not *be* at all. For this reason, the sun salutation is the very practice of consciousness and awareness itself. Moreover, in yoga, this light comes from the sun, the energy of the Earth, and in the salutation we accept, recognize, and receive the light from the sun, and we do so in order to awaken our own inner light.

Most of us, of course, probably practice our sun salutations indoors, at a gym or at a studio, so we do not actually receive the sunlight directly.

MEGAN M. BURKE

But this does not mean we do not receive light because our practice of this pose is focused on our relation to the sun: I open my chest, gaze upwards, and reach my arms above my head to welcome the sun, I inhale deeply to receive the sun's gift, and I do all of this with strength, commitment, and grace. It is, however, the case that my practice of the poses is strong when my intention to the sun is strong. I must direct my arms, my chest, and my gaze with a purpose to the sun. In this sense, it is the act of relating my self to the sun that matters here. A strong and graceful *surya namaskar* entails that one's intention and relation to the sun are strong and affirmed. When this happens, I welcome in and recognize the light and the energy of the Earth.

In order to use the light one creates in one's yoga practice, however, one needs a strong heart, and this strong heart comes from *ustrasana*, or camel pose. *Ustrasana* is a physically and emotionally difficult pose – the first time I did it, I was nauseous, I had tears rolling out of my eyes, and I thought I was going to pass out. But, as many of us know, it reaps some of the best benefits of any yoga pose: it stretches the stomach and intestines, strengthens our arms and shoulders, increases spine flexibility, and is a corrective for high blood pressure, among many other things. But *ustrasana* also does something else: it opens and strengthens our hearts. As I become a camel in this pose, I am vulnerable to the Earth and the environment around me, and, in so doing, I strengthen my humility because my vulnerability is a sign that I am a part of my surroundings. In my camel pose, I have the courage to bear my heart to the world and recognize my dependency on my environment. However, we also have the opportunity to do this on a daily basis outside of a yoga practice. While we spend much of our time trying to protect our vulnerability by building shelter, wearing clothing, buying insurance, and so on, we rarely consider why we do all of these actions. But, is it really insurance or clothing that will nourish life, or is there something more fundamental in the relationship between the Earth and ourselves that we must protect? In becoming a camel, my relationship to my surroundings changes; while posing like a camel, I feel and sense that I do not stand only on my own: I am connected to the Earth.

This recognition of a bond between my self and the environment also occurs in tree pose (*vrksasana*). Tree pose entails standing tall, firm, and proud like a healthy tree. One's legs become the trunk and one's arms the branches. One's center is firm and one's eyes gaze in meditation. While strength and steadiness of body and mind are found here, doing this pose in a world driven by deforestation is a powerful act of resistance.

Since tree pose requires yogis to honor the energy of the tree, yogis should protect trees and secure their livelihood off the yoga mat in order to receive and recognize their energy on the mat. *Vrksasana* can thus lead to an environmental consciousness.

Of course, these poses could be done without calling them by their names and the benefits might still be the same. But a genuine yoga practice recognizes the important connection between the name of the pose and the significance and benefits of the pose itself. When I am in the frog pose (*bhekasana*), it is not that I am a frog but that, in assuming the shape of a frog, I begin to relate to myself differently. In turn, I get a different perspective on the world. My frog-self feels differently than my camel-self and this feeling is a new practice of being myself. Rabbit pose (*sasangasana*), tree pose (*vriksasana*), eagle pose (*garudasana*), crow pose (*bakasana*), locust pose (*shalabhasana*), cat pose (*bidalasana*), and mountain pose (*tadasana*), among the many other poses named after non-human life forms, are meant to give yogis the strength and awareness of, and intention toward, the natural world. Yoga, meaning 'unity,' is, as the name suggests, a joining together: my self with nature. This union is a means to becoming different.

Asanas as Earth Democracy in Practice

In Shiva's book *Earth Democracy: Justice, Sustainability, and Peace*, she articulates ten principles of Earth democracy. Three of these principles, though arguably more, are at work in the practice of yoga's *asanas*. Two are 'Earth democracy is based on living cultures' and 'living cultures are life nourishing.' For Shiva, 'living cultures promote peace and create free spaces for the practice of different religions and the adoption of different faiths and identities' and this means Earth democracy is 'based on the dignity of and respect for all life, human and non-human, people of all genders and cultures.'[2] In other words, Earth democracy is an affirmation of life, a respect for living, and a commitment to promoting life and its diversity. Ultimately, these two principles result in practices and knowledge that affirm living processes and contribute to the health of the planet and people.

Yogis are attuned to this type of knowledge in the very moments of our *asanas*. Connecting with the life of other creatures – their strength, awareness, and postures in the world – is a means for each yogi to gain

MEGAN M. BURKE

new knowledge. Because *asanas* get us out of our habitual way of being in the world as soon as we take on the 'pose' of another creature, we are presented with the possibility of new knowledge. Standing as a tree, I can access insights that are unavailable to me when I stand in the checkout line at the grocery store. But, more importantly, the significance of this new knowledge when understood from Shiva's framework of Earth democracy is that it is fundamentally grounded in life: the new perspective offered in an *asana* emerges from a living entity that is different from me. Because of this, the newness that comes from an *asana* maintains and renews living processes.

The third principle of Earth democracy that is intimately related to yoga's *asanas* is the tenth: 'globalizing peace, care, and compassion.' For Shiva, this principle 'connects people in circles of care, cooperation and compassion instead of dividing them through competition and conflict,' and it 'globalizes compassion, justice, and sustainability.'[3] While it is a principle of non-violence, it also asserts that all of us are connected to one another such that our actions can lead to care or to war. This means that we must take an active role in deciding how we will act with others and with our environment. This is wisdom we gain directly from the practice of *asanas*. Because *asanas* shift our perspective, the practice itself reveals to us that we can feel, experience, and simply be other than what we currently are. If our current existence is characterized by fundamental negativity – that is, a destruction of the environment – then the practice of *asanas* allows us to both recognize this character and change it. The practice of *asanas* can lead us from war to care, from destruction to responsibility.

Understanding the practice of *asanas* in light of these two principles of Earth democracy reveals the practice itself as a transformative act of critique and an environmental ethic of care. Practicing *asanas* allows us to become different in our affirmation of living processes and, consequently, requires us to reflect on our current 'pose' or way of living in the world through taking on the pose of another life form. This becoming different through *asanas* leads to a critical awareness of our current place in the world, and lastly, with this critical awareness yogis generate a care between self and environment. Ultimately, we learn to care for life. We learn to care for and respect the life of the frog, the rabbit, the camel, the tree, the mountain, and our own life. Therefore, in our practice of *asanas* we gain a life- and Earth-affirming perspective, which is fundamental to an environmental ethic. In this sense, *asanas* as a practice of Earth democracy are not about giving Earth the right to vote, but recognizing that all life on Earth has a valuable perspective that should be both recognized and respected.

This connection between the yoga practice of *asanas* and Shiva's Earth democracy is even more plausible given that Shiva and yoga both deploy the Vedic notion, *vasudhaiva kutumbakam*, in their movements. *Vasudhaiva kutumbakam* asserts a primary and fundamental relationship between all living beings on Earth. As Shiva says in her book, the Sanskrit '*vasudhaiva kutumbakam*' means 'the Earth family'; it is 'the community of all beings supported by Earth.'[4] Taking this from the ancient spiritual scriptures of India, Shiva's Earth democracy is thus rooted in one of the fundamental tenets of yoga. As B. K. S. Iyengar says in *Astadala Yogamala, Volume 5*, 'The Earth is one family. The *Vedas* did not divide the Earth into parts.'[5]

For Iyengar, much like Shiva, the principle of *vasudhaiva kutumbakam* allows humans to acknowledge the continuity and connectedness between all beings on Earth. And more importantly, for Iyengar, yoga is one way to come to know *vasudhaiva kutumbakam*. He says, 'if yoga can build up the right knowledge, stabilize the emotions, transform instinct into intuition, take it from me that you and I lose all differences and we all become one. That is the universality of yoga.'[6] It is thus that, in becoming-frog or becoming-tree, the yogi loses her or his difference from the frog or the tree, and, given Shiva's and other environmentalists' assertions that the human relationship to nature is one of domination and a separation, transforming this relationship is a democratic practice for the Earth. In losing our separation from the Earth, through the very practice of *asanas*, we gain the wisdom of *vasudhaiva kutumbakam* and become, as Shiva says, 'members of the Earth community.'[7] This membership endows us with a 'duty to live in a manner that protects the Earth's ecological processes, and the rights and welfare of all species and all people.'[8]

Yogis for the Earth

Historically and philosophically, yoga has always asserted a fundamental metaphysical and ethical position in relation to nature. A concern for the environment, then, is central to the practice of yoga. From its very origins, yoga has not simply been a practice of meditation in nature, but has always asserted the continuity between humans and nature as its primary understanding of life. The practice of yoga is to remind us of this

MEGAN M. BURKE

continuity and the philosophy of yoga is to articulate it. Because of this, yoga's understanding of the relationship between humans and nature, which is embodied both in the philosophy behind the *asanas* and in the yogi herself as she practices them, is crucial to thinking about how we currently treat the Earth, in terms of both our immediate and global environments. As a yogi, I am for the Earth. But, recognizing the continuity between the Earth and myself is neither given nor easily ascertained through the *asanas*. Rather, each yogi needs to cultivate an awareness of her or his relationship and intentionality to nature that is embodied and articulated each time she or he becomes a frog, a rabbit, a camel, or a tree.

Furthermore, when she or he learns to appreciate and honor her or his relationship to the surrounding world through the *asanas*, she or he will be inclined to continue this practice off the mat. If *prana* matters to yoga, a yogi will think twice about the quality of air around her because she recognizes its significance to the continuation of life. If standing as a tree is a connection to trees, a yogi will not want to see trees bulldozed for new housing units. Or, in my case specifically, posing like non-human creatures revealed how little I think about non-humans in my typical human postures, such that I have developed great compassion for how non-humans are treated. Certainly, there are many other ways the practice of *asanas* leads to an environmental awareness. But, ultimately, the result is the same: yoga asks that we commit ourselves to actions that minimize environmental harm.

While *asanas* are only one step in a yogi's journey, their significance should not be undervalued or overlooked, especially when it comes to the connection they create between the yogi and the environment. Given the focus in Western culture on yoga's physical benefits, understanding the ethics behind the practice of *asanas* is significant. When I started practicing yoga, I never thought poses in which I became a camel, or a rabbit, or a tree, or saluting the sun would provide me with anything other than physical benefits. However, I came to realize that these physical benefits were secondary to much more gratifying, life-changing ones. Becoming non-human creatures in my poses has made me more aware of my intentions when I move off the mat. It is not that I have become a camel, or a frog, or a tree, but that I am learning to relate to the world through my own movements, my own posing in the world. And, I am learning to do this in connection with Earthly creatures that remind me of our integral connection to one another. For this reason, my yoga practice becomes a means of relating to the environment with openness and flexibility. These virtues are not merely physical benefits of yoga, but are a means to healing the human relationship with the environment.

NOTES

1 Vandana Shiva, 'The living democracy movement: Alternatives to the bankruptcy of globalization' (February 2003, http://www.zcommunications. org/the-living-democracy-movement-by-vandana2-shiva).

2 Vandana Shiva, *Earth Democracy: Justice, Sustainability, and Peace* (Cambridge, MA: South End Press, 2005), p. 11.

3 Ibid.

4 Ibid., p. 1.

5 B. K. S. Iyengar, *Astadala Yogamala, Volume 5* (New Dehli, India: Allied Publishers Private Limited, 2005), p. 87.

6 Ibid.

7 Shiva, *Earth Democracy*, p. 9.

8 Ibid.

MEGAN M. BURKE

CHAPTER 18

YOGA AND ETHICS
The Importance of Practice

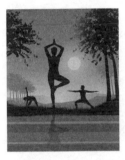

Introduction

Yoga and ethics are intrinsic to one another. That is to say, the purpose of yoga is essentially ethical and practicing ethics can be understood as yoga. In this essay I will endeavor to give some substance to this claim. However, the most convincing substantiation for me has come through yoga practice. It is through practicing yoga that I find an ease in living ethically in this world: in relating to those I am close to and in my interactions with others in my work-a-day world.

My interest in this topic is personal. By profession I am a teacher of ethics. I have been teaching ethics for the last twenty years (in three successive medical schools) and I am a yogi, having been practicing various forms of yoga for more than twenty years. Paradoxically, I believe that it is practicing yoga, rather than studying and teaching ethics, that has given me a better understanding of ethics – or at least a more practical and nuanced understanding.

Ethics in the West (with few exceptions) is identified with reason and the intellect rather than with practice. The emphasis in Western philosophy is on the question 'what is ethics?' and the professional response has been

Yoga – Philosophy for Everyone: Bending Mind and Body, First Edition.
Edited by Liz Stillwaggon Swan.
© 2012 John Wiley & Sons, Inc. Published 2012 by John Wiley & Sons, Inc.

to reason in terms of theories of ethics and codes of ethical behavior. Yet there is a gap between reason and practice. Knowing something to be true, or wise, or the right thing to do, is different from practicing it. And practicing a precept is a lot more challenging than acknowledging its wisdom.

As ethics has become more secular in the West, the emphasis has increasingly shifted to ethical reasoning and away from ethical practice. One consequence of a shift toward understanding ethics in terms of reasoning rather than practice is that Western scholars tend to look for the ethical content of yoga in yoga *texts* rather than in yoga *practice*.

The Role of Practice

It is by understanding yoga *through practice*, and *as practice*, that we can best understand the integral nature of ethics within yoga and find a deeper meaning of ethics in our lives. It is constant practice, rather than theory and reason, that is emphasized by yoga teachers.[1] Through immersing oneself in yoga and practicing its precepts, one gains an understanding of the intrinsic and integral place of ethics within the discipline. When this is not recognized, the tendency is to focus on yoga *texts* and to look for passages of text with recognizable ethical content. To limit our search in this way is to unconsciously import a Western bias and assumptions about ethics as being founded on reason. It gives too great a priority to texts, discourse, and words. This provides only a limited understanding and can trivialize ethics in yoga. What is written about ethics in yoga is most often a guide to practice and is not meant as a comprehensive theory of ethics. Focusing on texts, without engaging in the practice, diverts us from a richer understanding of the ethical import of yoga and circumvents a potential for yoga ethics to challenge and enrich Western ethics.

Yoga Scholarship

Many writers discussing yoga and ethics identify the moral disciplines (*yamas*) as the ethical precepts of yoga. There are ten *yamas* in various yoga texts including Yogi Swatmaram's *Hatha Yoga Pradipika* (fifteenth

PAUL ULHAS MACNEILL

century CE) and the *Yoga Sutras* of Patañjali (written sometime between 100 BCE and 500 CE). Although the particular disciplines (*yamas*) may differ from one list to another, most include non-violence (*ahimsa*), truthfulness (*satya*), non-stealing (*asteya*), non-coveting (*aparigraha*), and sexual responsibility (*brahmacharya*). Some (such as Patañjali's *Yoga Sutras*) include duties or observances (*niyamas*) such as purity and cleanliness (*saucha*), the practice of contentment (*santosha*), and self-discipline in the sense of practicing austerities (*tapas*). However, any tendency to identify yoga ethics with these *yamas* and *niyamas* overemphasizes their moral role and diminishes and distorts yoga ethics.

It is easy to see why the *yamas* and *niyamas* are presented as yoga ethics. Patañjali describes them as the first and second of eight 'limbs' or 'rungs' of yoga (*astav angani*). Some have taken this to indicate that the disciplines should be practiced as the first steps (or 'rungs') before moving on to yoga's other limbs in sequence (although Venkateshananda comments that 'these limbs should all be practised together').[2] Another reason that the *yamas* and *niyamas* are seen as yoga ethics is that they are often written (in translation) in the form of moral precepts and described as 'yoga's ten commandments.'

The *yamas* and *niyamas* are not, however, a complete system of ethics. They do not deal with larger questions such as 'why should one be ethical?' It is also apparent that many of them are not necessarily about ethics. One could make a case for why it is necessary for others that one should maintain purity and cleanliness, or practice contentment, but it is not obvious that anyone else is benefitted by those practices. This becomes even more apparent if we consider another two of Patañjali's *niyamas*: self-study or spiritual self-education (*svadhyaya*), and devotion to the supreme being (*ishvara pranidhanani*). It is hard to make the case that these are ethical precepts without understanding their place in the broader system. For this reason it is helpful to see how the *yamas* and *niyamas* fit within the broader context of Patañjali's *Yoga Sutras*.

Patañjali's *Yoga Sutras* have four chapters. The first is about *samadhi* – how to attain a state of 'uninterrupted self-awareness … peace and bliss.'[3] This is the attainment of yoga.[4] The first chapter offers a number of approaches to directly realizing this goal. However, if the reader is unable to directly experience *samadhi* (also described as 'enlightenment'), there is a second chapter that offers the *yamas* and *niyamas* as 'counter-measures' for overcoming 'the elements that cause mental turmoil' so as to turn 'one's attention towards enlightenment.'[5] Chapter 3 is about the nature of the mind, the causes of suffering, and freedom from desire (*vairagya*). The fourth chapter gives counsel on freeing the mind from false and imaginary notions of self and offers practices of meditation for doing so.

My point here is that identifying Patañjali's *yamas* and *niyamas* as yoga ethics, without placing them in the context of a practice designed to attain *samadhi*, is to misconstrue yoga and to give an impoverished view of yoga ethics. When they are understood in their context, it is clear that the *yamas* and *niyamas* are designed to lead to an end (*samadhi* – enlightenment), and they require practice in order to achieve that end. They are not necessarily *moral* edicts as such.

Aristotelian and Yoga Ethics

There are parallels between Patañjali's use of the *yamas* and *niyamas* and Aristotle's virtues in that both are designed to attain a goal (*telos*). Practicing Aristotelian virtues and acting in accordance with reason is a means to achieve the goal of happiness (*eudaimonia*). There are, however, major differences between *samadhi* and *eudaimonia*, and between the means by which yoga prepares the seeker for *samadhi*[6] and the means Aristotle advises for achieving *eudaimonia*. For Aristotle, ethics requires the application of practical reason (*phronesis*) to situations. Practice is needed to develop virtuous habits in order to become a virtuous person. The priority given to reason in Aristotelian ethics, however, is not evident in yoga. On the contrary, the goal of yoga is conceived as being beyond the understanding of reason and the discursive mind. Reason plays an important part, but it does not have the centrality that it is given in Aristotelian ethics. These are comparisons that warrant further exploration, but it is sufficient here to point to a common emphasis on the need for practice in both Aristotelian ethics and yoga, and to a *teleological* (goal-oriented) role in both systems for virtues and disciplines.

For Aristotle, the aim of life was happiness or *eudaimonia*, whereas in yoga it is described as *samadhi*, or self-realization. For this reason, both yoga and Aristotelian ethics have been portrayed as 'selfish,' or at least 'self-indulgent,' in that the apparent role of morality or virtue is self-serving. *Eudaimonia* is described as a natural inclination in all human beings, and a fulfillment of the purpose of life. While it has significance for the individual, it is not of itself of any necessary benefit to anyone else. Aristotelians could respond, however, that the virtues were

PAUL ULHAS MACNEILL

recommended for their own sake, not just as a means to happiness, and that a virtuous person (whether or not she attains happiness) would treat others well from a love of virtue.[7] Yoga's answer is that *samadhi* (or *self*-realization) *does* benefit others. Yogis claim that the experience is accompanied by a natural flow of compassion. This is a claim that is consistent with yoga metaphysics (which are discussed in the following two sections).

Yoga and Yoga Metaphysics

One of the criticisms that could be leveled against the position I am advancing is that I am using the word 'yoga' too inclusively. 'Yoga' is a word that has historically and culturally covered many different philosophies and practices. If yoga and ethics are to be regarded as intrinsic to each other – as I contend they are – then which 'yoga' is it that I am referring to? And, if I mean to include them all, in what way is ethics to be understood when each 'school' of yoga advances a somewhat different understanding of ethics? I address these questions by describing some of the different forms of yoga and saying how it is that I understand that yoga practice transcends these differences.

Yoga includes the practices of meditation; contemplation and self-study (*svadhyaya*); chanting; and devotional practices. It also includes *seva* (usually defined as 'selfless service'), physical postures (known as *asanas*) and breathing techniques (*pranayama*). These last two (*asanas* and *pranayama*) are together included within Hatha yoga, and are what is usually understood by 'yoga,' or 'Hatha yoga,' in the West. Typically a Hatha yoga practice includes standing postures; inverted poses (hand stands, head stands, and shoulder stands); forward bends, twists, and backbends; and at least one restorative pose (such as *shavasana*) to complete a session. In practicing *asana*, movements are usually coordinated with the breath. A practice session may also include *pranayama* and meditation.

In India, however, yoga is taken to include all these practices, and more. In some contexts the word 'yoga' is synonymous with 'Hinduism.' In the context of Indian philosophy, the word 'yoga' often denotes 'Samkhya yoga' – one of the six orthodox Hindu schools (*darshanas*, literally 'views') that are based on the *Vedas* (the ancient and revered Indian scriptures). In other contexts yoga is associated with particular

Indian texts (or scriptures), especially Patañjali's *Yoga Sutras*, Yogi Swatmaram's *Hatha Yoga Pradipika* (both mentioned above), and the *Bhagavad Gita*, an Indian religious text well known for its discussion of ethics. Each of these texts has its particular representation of yoga and its own ethical emphasis.

In this chapter I am using the word 'yoga' to include the practices of meditation, *asana*, and *pranayama* as well as yoga philosophy without limiting this philosophy to either Samkhya yoga or Patañjali's *Yoga Sutras* (as some do). Yoga has been enriched by the later school of Vedanta (especially Advaita Vedanta) and the philosophy of North Indian Kashmir Shaivism (not one of the orthodox *darshanas*), which I will discuss below.

Encompassing all these philosophies and religions, with their seemingly contradictory precepts, may seem to be overly inclusive (both to a naïve reader and to many scholars of Indian philosophy and religion). It is, however, consistent with the position I am developing: that an understanding of yoga and ethics transcends the limitations of any one philosophical system. An adequate understanding will only come through practice. It is through practice that many of the seeming paradoxes dissolve into an experience that transcends any one description. These various approaches can be understood as different ways of guiding the novice seeker to a full experience of yoga, and an understanding that encompasses many different views and descriptions of 'reality.' The differences between these systems then appear as the result of limitations of their discursive frame or textual nature, not as insuperable conflicts in and of themselves.

For examples of different portrayals of yoga (or Hindu) metaphysics, I draw on two of the later schools of Indian philosophy: Vedanta (particularly Advaita Vedanta) and Kashmir Shaivism (both mentioned above). The former portrays the world as unreal and Brahman (the supreme reality encompassing all that exists) as real. Our suffering results from attachment to the illusion (*maya*) that veils this transcendent reality. To practice in Vedanta is to continually challenge the limited notions of one's self, and its identity with a perceived and illusory world, in order to affirm one's identity with Brahman. By contrast, Kashmir Shaivism regards the world and everything in it as a manifestation of divine energy (or *sakti*) and as ultimately 'real.' Our suffering results from a perception of ourselves as separate from this divinity and its magnificence. The separation itself is the result of embroilment in the clamor and drama of the world and forgetting, or ignoring, our 'true' nature as divine energy. To practice in Kashmir Shaivism is to overcome this sense of separateness by identifying with divine energy so as to fully enjoy life in the world and a consequent flow of love and compassion between oneself and others.

Interestingly, although their metaphysics appear to be diametrically opposed, these practices amount to the same thing: an identification with (in the one case) a transcendent 'reality' that is both beyond and encompasses the 'illusory' world and (in the other) an identification with an imminent and expansive 'reality' of pulsing energy. While I have a preference for the metaphysics of Kashmir Shaivism – in that it affirms embodiment and this world as real – there are times, in the practice of meditation, when my experience could be described as transcendent (in the sense of transcending my body and physical circumstances). It is as if a realm, which far exceeds anything I ordinarily experience, opens to me. All is still, as if there is only *existence* itself. Even body awareness is lost to a powerful experience of stillness and transcendence. The temptation then is to describe ordinary existence, by comparison, as unreal or a mere shadow of this more expansive 'reality.' Alternatively, the experience in meditation can, at times, be one of a thrilling and earthy embodiment in which currents of energy are felt to enliven and illuminate every bodily movement and sensation. It is as if I am balanced on a knife edge of heightened alertness, excitement, and responsiveness to any slight current of change: a breeze touching my arm, a distant sound of a dog barking, or a tickle of energy moving inside my body. I feel so expanded that 'I' am both that dog barking and the sensation on my arm.

These experiences, one of transcendence and the other of immanence, are openings to something larger and more expansive than the everyday 'small self' going about its business as if with blinkers on. They are tastings, or samples, indicating that it may be possible to live in expanded awareness. The point of the metaphysics, whether it be Vedantan or Kashmir Shaivite, is to direct each of us to this expansiveness. The metaphysical systems, in and of themselves, are neither true nor false. They serve as instruments in attaining the goal of yoga, which is to live in a constant experience of expanded awareness, inner harmony, and uninterrupted joy. Yogis have given this experience various names, including *samadhi* and self-realization. The various names denote a *locus* of experience beyond the 'small self' and identified with universal energy, Brahman, or Self (with a capital 's'), that encompasses all people and all sentient beings.

Yoga and Ethics

Nisargadatta Maharaj (1897 to 1981) was a yogi (spiritual teacher) who lived in Bombay. He said that 'one who is devoted to his own Self becomes the soul of all. Who, then, will have ill will and for whom? One becomes helpful to others naturally knowing that one is not different from them.'[8] Inherent in this teaching is a metaphysics in which the small self is dissolved, through yogic practice, into the universal Self. There one experiences that 'charity and love are naturally present.'[9] In a similar vein, John Friend (author of the "Foreword" of this book) describes the ethics of yoga as flowing from an intention 'to glorify *Shri*' – which is translated as 'that which is life-enhancing, beautiful, and auspicious.' Ethics, then, rather than being imposed, derives from practices that support an expansive and 'life-enhancing' vision of oneself 'as a divine being full of goodness and greatness.'[10]

The metaphysics (as belief structures) are not of primary importance here. Yoga metaphysics are a support for practicing yoga. Following (and sometimes during) practice, there may be glimpses of change: a flow of greater compassion; a surprising moment of generosity toward someone in unexpected circumstances; and living one's life in less pain, and with increasingly frequent moments of joy. These are indications that give some cogency to the chosen metaphysics, regardless of the system one is working with.

As indicated above, yoga comprises many different practices, including meditation and self-study (or self-attentiveness), that help to dissolve a sense of 'I am' as separate from everyone else. From this dissolution of self, in Nisargadatta's words, 'compassion will flow through you.'[11] This is the foundation of yoga ethics: that when we realize our expanded nature, even to a small extent, we are naturally inclined to treat others well.

While yoga precepts and moral restraints support ethical behavior, they are not themselves the substance – and certainly not the extent – of yoga ethics. As stated at the outset, ethics is intrinsic to yoga and it is in this sense that we look for ethics within yoga's metaphysics, core objective, and practices. More convincing, however, is that, in practicing yoga and working toward the goal of self-realization, we naturally become more ethical, not from duty but from inclination. This is because we discover (or recognize) ourselves to be one – or at least 'at one' – with others, not as a belief, but as a powerful and convincing experience. These realizations

PAUL ULHAS MACNEILL

can also happen the other way around. By practicing ethical virtues (e.g., compassion, generosity, forbearance, and restraint with others) one can experience oneself as more expansive. It is in this sense that practicing ethics can be understood as yoga (as I claimed at the outset).

Why Hatha Yoga?

The link between ethics and the practices of meditation and contemplation is more readily apparent than the link between ethics and the practice of yoga postures and breathing techniques. There is a certain 'face validity' to claims that meditation and contemplation can assist one in dealing with a fractious mind and intemperate behavior toward others. So the question remains: how do the physical postures (*asana*) and breath control (*pranayama*) contribute to becoming a more compassionate and ethical person? To answer this question I refer to B. K. S. Iyengar, a well-known Indian yoga master and an accepted authority on Hatha yoga in both India and the West. Iyengar gives several reasons for practicing yoga *asana*:

> Asana brings steadiness, health and lightness of limb ... [It] produces mental equilibrium and prevents fickleness of mind ... It is a state of complete equilibrium of body, mind and spirit. ... The yogi frees himself of physical disabilities and mental distractions by practicing asanas.[12]

Iyengar claims that there is a relationship between breath, mind, and spirit. This is relatively easy to observe: an agitated mind and emotional excitement 'affect the rate of breathing.' Conversely, by regulating the breath, 'the heart will be at peace.' The practice of *pranayama* establishes 'proper rhythmic patterns of slow deep breathing' and prepares the yogi for concentration and meditation.[13]

These benefits from *asana* and *pranayama* also relate to ethics and ethical behavior in that (from the perspective of yoga) ethical behavior is the 'natural' expression of a person in equilibrium. What Hatha yoga addresses is some of the distortions that create *dis*equilibrium.

All of us accumulate distortions of various kinds that manifest physically as postural habits or as misalignments in the body. Distortions and agitations of mind manifest as anxiety and other disturbances. These make it difficult to function in a flowing and graceful manner. They need to be addressed in the body and mind, and yoga is an effective means for doing that. Anthropologist Michael Jackson, for example, described his early practice of yoga (in his mid-thirties) as 'unpicking the locks of a cage.' He added that:

> I began to live my body in full awareness for the first time, feeling the breath, under my conscious control, fill my lungs, experiencing through extensions and *asanas* the embodied character of my will and consciousness. ... [This] transformed awareness brought me up against the full force of habit, of set attitudes and ingrained dispositions. It quickly became clear to me that dystonic habits of body use cannot be changed by desiring to act in different ways.[14]

The point Jackson makes about desiring to act in different ways is especially pertinent to this discussion of ethics. It takes more than desire to address 'the full force of habit ... set attitudes and ingrained dispositions.' It is in working with the body and mind in a disciplined way that these patterns may be revealed and dissolved.

An inner gaze

Yoga practice includes a particular focus on working with the body to free oneself from 'ingrained dispositions.' Practitioners are encouraged to maintain a gaze that is both external *and* turned inward: as though one is looking both externally and internally at the same time. This is to practice yoga being aware of one's body and one's surroundings, *and* focusing on one's inner experience simultaneously. This gaze is known as *sambhavi mudra*. It is a gaze in which the yoga student both looks and is aware of herself looking. It is said that, without that inner attention, yoga postures cannot be called yoga. They are simply physical exercises. Iyengar puts forward a similar idea, albeit in more 'religious' terms, in stating that 'true *asana* is that in which the thought of Brahman flows effortlessly and incessantly through the mind of the *sadhaka*.'[15]

Discussion

I venture to claim that none of these recognitions about ethics in yoga would have been open to me without a committed yoga practice. Yoga philosophy was initially exciting and enticing, but when I read from

PAUL ULHAS MACNEILL

different sources I was lost in conflicting and discordant messages. Through a consistent practice, these conflicts no longer trouble me. I see them as apparent rather than real, and as different approaches to an experience that is unreachable through words alone. However, it has been slow work, in different corners of yoga, stretching over three decades.

Although this essay is about yoga and ethics, the point about understanding through practice is also valid for other Asian disciplines. On the basis of my earlier efforts (prior to practicing yoga) in Japanese martial arts (judo, jujitsu, and karate), Buddhist meditation, and Tai Chi, I maintain that these claims about the importance of practice are also true for many other Asian disciplines and practices.

Furthermore, the understanding I have gained about ethics through all these practices is more subtle than any understanding open to me through studying and teaching Western ethics. There is an elusive quality about relating ethically that is more of the nature of art than science – a flowing, an elegance, that is more poetry than prose. It may be that artists and musicians have a similar experience in that their art is similarly elusive. This quality can be found in one's relationships, communication, and sensitivity to others. There may be some basic things that can be said about it, but the quality I am referring to evades description. What can be said is that acting and living ethically require practice and constant fine attention to the effects of our words, actions, and silences both on others and within ourselves.

It alarms me, however, that ethics in the West, at least in the professions and academia, is largely about theory and ethical principles. In any of the arts this would signal a low level of development, like a dancer attempting to move with a diagram of the basic steps in hand. Anyone who can dance has long ago thrown away the guidebook. But, in the professions – even in medicine, which is surely about practice and relationship – the talk is about theory, principles, and guidelines, and very little of it focuses on ethics as practice. This is not to deny that physicians do indeed practice ethics. However, with few exceptions,[16] there is little discussion of a nuanced understanding of practicing one's discipline with ethics, and compassion for others, as intrinsic and integral to the discipline itself.

An understanding of ethics – as intrinsic to practicing yoga and to attaining fulfillment in life – can challenge and enrich Western ethics. In this, and many other respects, yoga has much to offer us.

Acknowledgements

An earlier oral version of this paper was presented at the 9th World Congress of Bioethics in Rijeka, September 2008. I am grateful to the congress organizers, and particularly Dr. Iva Sorta-Bilajac, for the opportunity to develop and present these ideas.

I appreciate many insights gained from Dr. Carlos G. Pomeda's video lecture series on yoga philosophy, and particularly his attention to a 'sequential' reading of the chapters of Patañjali's *Yoga Sutras*, in terms of prioritizing their importance (as discussed in the section entitled 'Yoga Scholarship').

I am grateful to my many teachers on the path of yoga for their patience, compassion, and unstinting generosity in supporting my practice and tentative steps toward understanding. While there are too many to name them all, I acknowledge in particular, and with gratitude, love, and respect: Mr George Adie, Baba Muktananda, Swami Venkateshananda, Swami Ranganathananda, Gurumayi Chidvilasananda, John Friend, Craig Sharp, Swami Anantananda, Sally Kempton, and Dr. Carlos G. Pomeda.

NOTES

1   B. K. S. Iyengar, *Light on Yoga* (New York: Schocken Books, 1977).

2   Swami Venkateshananda, *Enlightened Living: A New Interpretative Translation of The Yoga Sutra of Maharṣi Patañjali* (Elgin Cape Province, South Africa: The Chiltern Yoga Trust, 1975), Sutra II.29. Also available online: http://www.swamivenkatesananda.org/clientuploads/publications_online/Enlightened%20Living%20by%20Swami%20Venkatesananda.pdf.

3   Ibid., Sutra I.47.

4   Ibid., Sutra I.2.

5   Ibid., Sutras II.2 and II.33.

6   Ibid., at Sutra II.2.

7   M. F. Burnyeat, 'Aristotle on learning to be good.' In A. O. Rorty (Ed.), *Essays on Aristotle's Ethics* (Berkeley and Los Angeles, CA: University of California Press, 1980), pp. 69–92.

8   Matthew Greenblatt (Ed.), *The Wisdom Teachings of Nisargadatta Maharaj* (Carlsbad, CA: Inner Directions, 2003), p. 73.

9   Ibid., p. 83.

10 'Ethics,' *Anusara* (n.d., http://www.anusara.com/index.php?option=com_content&view=article&id=133&Itemid=185).

PAUL ULHAS MACNEILL

11 Greenblatt, *The Wisdom Teachings of Nisargadatta Maharaj*, p. 56.
12 Iyengar, *Light on Yoga*, pp. 40–41.
13 Ibid., pp. 43–45.
14 Michael Jackson, *Paths Toward a Clearing: Radical Empiricism and Ethnographic Inquiry* (Bloomington, IN: Indiana University Press, 1989), p. 119.
15 Iyengar, *Light on Yoga*, p. 42.
16 Paul A. Komesaroff, *Experiments in Love and Death: Medicine, Postmodernism, Microethics and the Body* (Melbourne, Australia: Melbourne University Press, 2008).

CHAPTER 19

WHY ARE YOU STANDING ON MY YOGA MAT?!

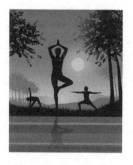

Most people's behaviors and conscious thoughts reveal a preoccupation with themselves – desires for success, esteem, love, and creature comforts. However, deep within seemingly selfish individuals there is often a 'hidden ethical self' waiting to be revealed. Ordinary human beings perform acts of extraordinary self-sacrifice when this ethical self is activated. Emergencies awaken it, as with the firemen who bravely worked around the clock to remove bodies from the rubble of the 9/11 attacks. However, none of us is forced to wait for an urgent situation to awaken our hidden ethical selves. Both philosophical arguments and spiritual experiences can excite the hidden ethical self to lifelong action. There are good philosophical reasons to show that, if you care about yourself, you should also care about others. Yoga, likewise, through experience rather than argument, can move a person from selfishness to caring about others.

The yogic path is one that unlocks our unconsciously held beliefs, awakens our deepest ethics, and helps us to live in harmony with ourselves, others, and the environment. Yoga (meaning 'union') is concerned with uniting a person's body and mind (through breath, awareness, and

Yoga – Philosophy for Everyone: Bending Mind and Body, First Edition.
Edited by Liz Stillwaggon Swan.
© 2012 John Wiley & Sons, Inc. Published 2012 by John Wiley & Sons, Inc.

movement).The natural development of a devoted practice is an alignment of the person's actions with her highest values, promoting personal integrity and often concern for others and the environment as well. Such a yogic practice produces a naturally satisfying, centered, and ethical life.

This essay offers a series of philosophical arguments and complimentary yoga exercises that are intended to awaken your deepest personal ethics to help you understand and care more for yourself, others, and the environment. The yoga exercises include movement (*asana*), breathing (*pranayama*), and meditation (*dhyana*).

The first section focuses on removing obstacles in ourselves that prevent us from being whole and ethical. The second presents three arguments that demonstrate how one's self-discovery can unearth natural and rational care for others and the environment.

Uncovering the Whole Self for Integrity in Action

Self-exploration as a prerequisite for caring for others

It is natural for us to perceive a difference between ourselves and others. However, in deep, clear-minded, philosophical reflection, it is just as natural for us to recognize that others are an extension of the self. Philosophical arguments and yoga practice can reinforce each other and help us to care more deeply for others and the environment. In an argument that helps to uncover our hidden ethical selves, it makes sense to seek first a better understanding of ourselves. What defines me? Who am I? Am I realizing my full potential? Without the ability to see who we are, we will be unable to see others for who they are. How can we be loving, respectful, and compassionate if we do not understand the individuals we are trying to care for?

Exercise 1: *Asana* for basic self-awareness

In flowing and simple *asana*, the body is a gateway to the mind, preparing the mind for self-discovery. Breathing deeply and exhaling completely in union with the movements increases the benefits of *asana* practice. Focused breathing in *asana* interrupts obsessive-compulsive thinking associated with unproductive mental patterns. This enables us to confront our problems (instead of simply dwelling on them) and live with more peace of mind.

A simple *asana* practice for self-awareness begins with closing the eyes and moving through a series of flowing movements. The mind observes the changes in the body that take place during the dynamic movement and the mind attunes itself to it. One might do neck and shoulder rolls and arm stretches. Other yogis might prefer sun salutations.

As yoga practitioners know, *asana* is insufficient for self-transformation. It is one of the most effective preparations, however, for deeper reflection and meditation, both of which will be the focus of the remaining exercises.

Seeking the whole self: Roles

An exploration of the self begins with an inquiry into who you are. You may be a son or daughter; Irish, Mexican, or Vietnamese; Hindi, Muslim, or atheist. You may be a yogi, an academic, or an artist. You may love the ocean, the mountains, or the city. You may aspire to do the perfect handstand, to be a vegetarian, or to run regularly. You may shun categorization entirely, but of course you also know that this very attitude is also part of what defines you.

People have various roles they play and goals they hope to accomplish. Some roles we inherit simply in virtue of being born to certain people in a certain place at a certain time. We also have roles we have chosen to some degree or another. Our goals spring from these roles and our attitudes toward them, whether we stoically accept them, enthusiastically embrace them, or vehemently rebel against them.

When our roles are conscious, we may call them conceptions of ourselves. These conceptions produce our beliefs, help to create our desires, and spur us to action. We may also inhabit roles of which we are not fully aware. For example, a woman may unconsciously consider herself to have a defect. She may not fully realize that her discontent with herself is dependent upon an unconsciously held belief of how women should be (beautiful, with a significant other, having children). Deeply exploring ourselves enables us to assess and revise our strategies in life that may not be working.

Exercise 2: Writing meditation – What are my roles?

In writing meditation, the hand is an extension of the mind, allowing the mind to freely, though concretely, express itself though the movements of the body. It brings to light unconscious thoughts. Write everything that you are currently thinking without censoring yourself. Many find it helpful to use a pen and paper rather than a computer, since the movements are more organic and allow for a wider range of possible writings, including drawing. Writing meditation also provides a basis for deeper reflection.

Ask yourself: What are my roles? Which activities express who I am? What are my goals? You may find it helpful to begin your writing meditation simply with the words 'I am a' and later with 'I love,' 'I enjoy,' and 'I want.'

Multiple roles and conflicts

We have a multiplicity of roles. These ways of being and our reactions to them, conscious or not, constitute who we are and how we are seen. We might call the whole of a person's roles, aspirations, and attitudes toward those roles and desires that person's practical identity as an individual.[1]

In our journey to discover ourselves we see that our present struggles are only small instances of thematic lifelong challenges we face. Our thematic struggles emerge from conflicts within our identities. There are two basic kinds of conflict in our identities and aspirations. There are practical conflicts, such as the inability to afford something you greatly desire or the inability to do everything you dream of because of job and family limitations. And then there are theoretical conflicts, between roles that are to some degree irreconcilable in principle, such as being a soldier and a pacifist or a meat-eater and an advocate of animal rights. Both kinds of conflict call us to revise our conceptions of ourselves and consequently how we live our lives.

We can revise our practical identities to the extent that they are chosen. Even if a conception of oneself is inescapable (e.g., being a daughter), the expectations associated with that role can be assessed and revised. One way of evaluating whether a person's conception of herself is good asks whether and to what extent the conception satisfies her underlying reason for having it. How many of our identities, goals, and activities truly satisfy our purposes? Are they among the best to fulfill our purposes? Do some of them interfere with satisfying other goals that we have in ways that could be avoided?

Not all conceptions can be revised, nor all conflicts resolved. Sometimes we must come to grips with the ways in which our lives are messy. However, dealing with the revisable and reconcilable energizes us to focus on roles and aspirations that give the most meaning to our lives. We then have resources to better deal with those parts of us that remain in conflict. In conflict we need not always struggle.

Exercise 3: Insight meditation – What are my struggles?

Insight meditation begins when a person's mind is calm enough to begin going deeply into itself, observing its contents, attitudes, and processes. This kind of meditation can aid in discovery and resolution of conflicts between one's roles, ideals, expectations, and aspirations. Begin comfortably seated. Breathe deeply. It may help to relax each part of the body one by one in a method called 'progressive relaxation.' Give your intuition freedom to respond, uninhibited by the usual justifications the mind gives to defend (rather than expose) the self. Observe your immediate responses and acknowledge any resistance, feelings, or thoughts that emerge.

Ask yourself: What are my current life struggles? What beliefs about myself, others, and 'what ought to be' lie behind these struggles? Are these beliefs true? Breathe deeply and repeat a simple insight you learned before emerging from your meditative state. Your insight may be anything from a word or phrase, such as 'love and let go' to a sentence 'I have freedom to choose my own path.' Your words will arise naturally from your observations. Afterwards, write about your responses.

Exercise 4: Insight meditation – Am I struggling unnecessarily?

Reflect on your previous meditation. Ask yourself: Am I struggling unnecessarily? What belief or expectation could I release that would make me more free? Breathe deeply and allow your response to flow through your mind and body as a mantra. Whenever the struggles come to your mind, ask yourself the above questions, observe your answers, and allow an insight mantra to fill you as you breathe.

Reconciliation of roles: Uniting the whole self

So far, we have sought to reveal our roles and expectations, observed how they interact and where we struggle, and meditated on letting go of certain roles and beliefs in order to struggle less and create more freedom in ourselves. These philosophical and yogic explorations open greater self-awareness and less conflicted ways of being. However, a more complete unity in the self is possible. If we are able to grasp that certain roles and ways of being are more primary to ourselves and our well-being than others, we can begin to unite ourselves in ways that naturally resolve our personal and interpersonal conflicts. In appreciating our own greatest good, we lay the foundation for a deeper understanding and appreciation of others and their greatest good.

For example, many people seek material wealth without giving much thought to how it will serve their other needs and desires. Most people choose between competing jobs almost entirely on the basis of salary and then end up realizing that substantial other goods (location, loss of relationships from moving, and workplace atmosphere) should have been more prominent players in the decision-making process.[2] Conversely, if a person begins to see wealth as something that aids the attainment of happiness, she can begin to assess what makes her happy by introspection and observation of her responses to her experiences. She can begin to see that some roles and goals she chooses are a means to, or are part of, her, happiness. When two of her roles conflict, she can assess them in light of that awareness.

When we recognize that some roles are more central to our identities than others, we can re-evaluate the importance of our roles and revise or dismiss those that are inaccurate or not beneficial to our overall well-being. The roles that unify us with ourselves also unify us with others and the environment. This will emerge in three arguments in the second section of this essay.

Exercise 5: Insight meditation – What have I been seeking?

On the one hand, this meditation may be a way of intuitively uncovering your greater good from a place of personal insight. On the other hand, it may bring to your consciousness the revelation that you have been concentrating on something that is detrimental to your overall well-being.

After practicing *asana* and simple breathing for relaxation, ask yourself from a place of deep calm: What have I been seeking in life? What have I been neglecting? What do I need most right now? Respect your intuitive response and observe your reactions. Repeat your response to yourself, letting the benefits of your mental clarity and insight sink deeper into your consciousness.

Uncovering our bonds with others and the environment

After uniting ourselves through an exploration of our practical identities, uncovering our self-defeating roles, and revising those roles so they are more beneficial for us, we are in a better position to awaken our hidden ethical selves. Introspection into our practical identities and observations of our dependencies on our environments enable us to recognize and create deep bonds of caring between ourselves, all of humanity, and the world.

Natural and instinctive caring for others

Selfishness can prevent us from being ethical. We can help remove the obstacles by understanding the ways in which we are unselfish. One natural inclination that nearly all humans have is caring about their families. We sometimes go to extreme lengths, incurring deep financial and emotional burdens to help our families live long, healthy, and happy lives. Mothers give up career aspirations to care for their children. Siblings protect each other. Children devote themselves to caring for their aging parents. Why do we so naturally care about our families? We do not love them simply because they are loving, useful, or enjoyable to us, since we often love them in the absence of these benefits.

Our friends, neighbors, and those we interact with regularly also tend to occupy special places in our circle of concern. Deep bonds develop between people of different backgrounds, personalities, and values. These often appear to be traceable to living closely to one another in a community where our welfare is affected by others.

Exercise 6: Guided imagery meditation – My natural circle of concern

Prepare yourself for meditation by practicing *asana* and simple breathing to relax your body and mind. Close your eyes and imagine that you are in a beautiful, serene place. It may be a place that gave you comfort or inspiration in the past, or it may be your creation. Sit in your special place. Observe yourself and your surroundings in detail. You see a person in the distance. It is the person you love most in the world. See that person approaching you. Rise to greet your loved one and offer a seat beside you. As you two sit together, you observe more people approaching. They are all the people you care for deeply. Observe and greet your loved ones by name, offering each a seat beside you. Enjoy sitting beside them and observe your feelings. Breathe deeply with them in unison – slow, long, relaxing breaths. Smile at each person before you close your eyes in your special place and come back to your own solo breathing where you now sit in meditation.

Caring through a common interest or purpose

Common interests or goals also serve to ground natural caring between people. Friendships develop in academic environments when we realize that someone else likes something we like, such as poetry, biology, or political activism. For example, we might start investing in people who

HEATHER SALAZAR

play on our soccer team because we have to and then we end up caring about them in the process. Sharing activities and purposes with others gives us opportunities to open ourselves to others and take them into our circle of concern. Sometimes our common roles and aspirations lead more naturally to competitiveness. In these contexts, rather than investing in others' welfare, we invest in their demise, which we will explore next.

Exercise 7: Partner *asana* for connection and cooperation

In partner yoga two people connect to move and breathe as one. It is not simply doing yoga beside someone, but rather doing it as if you were one being. It teaches us to connect to another person instead of acting alone or competing. Ask a friend to join you in a partner *asana* practice. Begin by facing each other while standing. Look into the other person's eyes gently and steadily. Raise your hands in synchronicity as you lightly but firmly press your palms into your friend's palms. Move your hands in slow outward and then inward circles, taking care to not lead or rush your friend. Stop when it feels natural. Place your hands on each other's shoulders, close your eyes, and feel your friend's breathing. Breathe together.

Rationally and Naturally Moving beyond Selfishness

Argument 1: Extending our care to all of humanity

While natural forms of caring show us insights about ourselves and how caring is produced, natural forms of non-caring can be rationally exposed as instances of dysfunctional thinking. In recognizing that we have a common hobby with someone else, we must look deeper than the hobby itself to the reason we both have the hobby. In other words, the same method we used to dissolve conflicts in ourselves (from the section "Reconciliation of Roles: Uniting the Whole Self") can be enlisted to dissolve barriers between ourselves and others. When we ask ourselves why we are interested in studying philosophy, exhibiting art, or competing in a marathon, we see that we are motivated to do something active that we love or that brings us a sense of accomplishment, whether it be in seeking knowledge, creative expression, or making an impact on the world. And this commonality of reason that underlies our interests, aspirations, and roles is hardly superficial, as it unites us with *all of humanity*, no matter what each person's interests are. Though I may not share my neighbor's interest in running, I can see that it is valuable for her as a way to exert herself physically and feel empowered. I do not run, but I dance for similar reasons. Others may cook, mentor, or take long solo vacations.

In caring about people we need not endorse their particular interests. Playing video games might seem dull or unproductive to one person but to jump to the conclusion that it is an unworthy or bad activity misses the point. There might be unworthy or bad activities, but asking about a person's reasons delves deeper into the person. Why does the person like playing video games? What does she get from it? My friend explains the appeal of them to me as enabling her to create and compete in her own adventure. I can see the value of that because I read books and write stories for the same reason. We see that we are bonded to all others more through our reasons for why we do the things we do than the doing of the things themselves.

Similarly, people who compete with us, whether in a sporting event, for a job, or for a romantic partner, are doing what they love, desiring to put their passions into practice, and wanting a happy and fulfilled life, just like we are. Once we observe the reasons that link us, how can we fail to give others the same respect that we give ourselves and those we naturally care about? In sympathy of purpose we are bonded with others by human concerns.

This type of argument follows in the tradition of the philosopher Immanuel Kant. It enlists the recognition of our shared humanity to argue that we must value others in the same way we value ourselves. We would negate our own worth as people who have identities, values, and goals if we were to fail to see the worth in others' identities, values, and goals. If we are able to unify ourselves, then with a little additional reflection we can see how we are unified with others.

Exercise 8: Guided imagery for understanding and compassion

Sit comfortably and breathe deeply. Gently relax each part of your body. Imagine in detail a person with whom you are currently having a conflict. Invite the person to sit opposite you and say: 'What is troubling you? Please tell me and I will listen.' Don't try to solve the problem or reply with your opinion. Do you understand what is troubling the person? Tell the person so. Place your hands in prayer position by your heart and imagine a small glowing ball of heart energy between your palms. Observe it pulsating as you extend it to the person and smile. Ask: 'What would help to relieve your suffering?' Could you imagine helping the person? In a sense, you already have. Listening deeply with understanding to a person's troubles is itself a way to alleviate their suffering. In listening and understanding, we also reduce our own suffering. Instead of putting negative energy into reacting to the person and trying to get your way, you have stopped struggling. Breathe deeply and observe your reactions to the exercise.

Argument 2: Extending our care to animals, plants, and other living things

Kant argued that the recognition of our shared use of reasons entails that we have obligations to respect and value each other. Some people question Kant's assumption that animals lack reasons for their actions. However, we can sidestep these concerns and argue that we are obligated to respect all animals, plants, and other living things (regardless of whether they are rational or not). Neo-Kantian philosopher Christine Korsgaard uses the idea of practical identities to argue that we must recognize the value not only in other people but in all living things. If we value ourselves in certain ways, then we must value other things that exhibit traits that are similar to those we value in ourselves.

We, as people, have purposes for why we believe and do certain things. As we explored in the previous sections, people often have similar reasons for pursuing different kinds of activities. For example, we exercise because we want to be healthy. We pursue loving relationships because it makes us happy. We see value in living long, healthy, and happy lives. Our reasons link us, but so do our values. Animals can experience happiness. And all living things can experience health, growth, and longevity. We see value in these attributes and use them to justify our pursuits. Animals and other living things experience these goods, so we must value animals and other living things as well. Life and happiness matter to us, so we must recognize that they are valuable, regardless of whether they are in our own person, or in that of another person, animal, or plant.

Argument 3: Caring for others and the world as a way of caring for ourselves

My third argument for naturally and rationally extending our circle of concern stretches beyond caring for other humans, animals, and other living things. It entreats us to care about everything in the world. Furthermore, it approaches the topic from a different perspective, relying on a simple yet profound truth that some Buddhists call 'interdependence.'[3]

That we share the world with others is an inescapable fact of our existence. We share the environment and the community. We depend on others, whether the fire department, the farmer, or the bank, for our welfare. We depend on people economically for exchange and distribution of resources and services that affect our daily lives. The goods in our lives require a complex web of skilled people who produce and share knowledge, services, and products. And we depend on the land, the water, and the air (as well as everything in them). Trees beautify our parks and also provide the wood for homes, paper, and even fabric. The people, animals, and elements of our natural environments contribute substantially and often necessarily to our wellness, productivity, and recreation. Caring about them and their welfare *just is* a way for us to care about ourselves since we so deeply affect and rely on each other. It is responsible for us to affect others in a positive way, both for their welfare and for our own.

Exercise 9: Insight meditation – The world in a cup of tea

For this meditation you will need a small cup of tea. Closely observe the tea in your hands. Feel it against your hands, touch it to your lips, smell it, and slowly take a sip. Breathe deeply and relish all of the sensations that the tea provides. Your thirst is now one sip more quenched, your body one sip of tea more nourished. Imagine what it took to bring this cup of tea to you today. Besides the tea leaves, it took hot water, a pot, and a cup to put it in. It took electricity or gas and an appliance. The tea was grown and harvested by people who likely live very far from where you are now. The tea needed seeds, fertile soil, sun, and water from the earth. The metals, ceramic, and petroleum for the plastic and gas came from the earth. In as much detail as possible, imagine the processes and the people that it took to bring this cup of tea to you today. Many hundreds of people and many parts of the Earth cooperated in making this single cup of tea. Every time you sip a cup of tea, you can remember how the world – both its living and non-living inhabitants – played an integral role in its existence.

Conclusion

By uncovering our own identities and resolving barriers in ourselves, we unify ourselves under a greater good for our own welfare. In seeing the

HEATHER SALAZAR

connections between ourselves, others, and the environment, we uncover our hidden ethical selves, caring about others and the environment as a way of honoring ourselves, others, and our intimate interdependence.

NOTES

1   I have borrowed the term 'practical identity' from Christine Korsgaard (see particularly *The Sources of Normativity*, Cambridge, UK: Cambridge University Press, 1996). She has inspired some of my views on the subject of morality. In metaphysical reflection on the self in spiritual circles it is often said that there is no 'self' – no 'identity' – and that these concepts are illusions that keep us imprisoned within our egos. Note that the current exploration of individual identity is not in conflict with this greater spiritual view. The self in what Buddhists often call the 'relative realm' or the 'conditioned realm' is necessary for insight into the non-self in the 'universal realm' or the 'unconditioned realm.' See Thich Nhat Hanh's *The Heart of the Buddha's Teaching* (Berkley, CA: Parallax Press, 1998) for a particularly lucid description of the interdependence of the self and the non-self.

2   See Boris Groysberg and Robin Abrahams, 'Managing yourself: Five ways to bungle a job change,' *Harvard Business Review* (January–February 2010).

3   This concept is also related to the Buddhist ideas of emptiness and non-self, among others.

NOTES ON CONTRIBUTORS

JIM BERTI, when not performing downward dog, likes listening to 'Downward Dog' (by moe.) and stretching his mind to the music of Rush. When not on the yoga mat, Jim can be found in his classroom teaching eighth-graders at Shaker Junior High School how to find the 'balance' between homework and tests. He credits his yoga practice for his newfound respect of nature, and for his discovery of the untapped potential of the mind and body.

KEN BURAK is a philosophy professor at Northampton Community College in Pennsylvania; husband of Liz Wheeler, father of two girls, Hannah and Dhara; and author of *Logic and Resistance: Reading Hegel in the Age of the War on Terrorism* (VDM, 2005). He once asked Hannah, who is six, where she ended and the tree in front of her began. She answered: 'I begin at the line, and end at the circle.' He asked Dhara, who is four, whether her mind was using her body or her body was using her mind. She answered immediately: 'Both and both at the same time.' Woah…

MEGAN M. BURKE is a graduate student in philosophy at the University of Oregon, where she spends a lot of time thinking about human relationships with other living creatures, human and non-human. While in school, she spends most of her time perfecting the postures of

Yoga – Philosophy for Everyone: Bending Mind and Body, First Edition.
Edited by Liz Stillwaggon Swan.
© 2012 John Wiley & Sons, Inc. Published 2012 by John Wiley & Sons, Inc.

becoming-camel and becoming-rabbit in her yoga practice. She lives with her canine companion who has a graceful *adho mukha svanasana*.

LUNA DOLEZAL was born in Australia. She currently lives in Dublin with her cat Leo. Previously having studied physics and literary theory, Luna has turned to philosophy. She is currently completing her PhD at University College Dublin, Ireland (funded by the Irish Research Council for Humanities and Social Sciences). Luna started practicing yoga in 1998 and has now taught yoga for many years.

LEIGH DUFFY received her PhD in philosophy in 2009 from the University at Buffalo. After five very unbalanced years there, studying epistemology and writing a dissertation on 'modal illusions,' she finally found balance as a philosopher, teacher, and yogi. She then gave birth to a baby boy in 2010 and that newfound sense of balance was completely overthrown. Leigh alternates between dressing her son in a T-shirt that says 'Ask me about Modal Illusions' and one that says 'Namaste' to remind herself to keep balancing work, play, and parenthood.

NICOLE DUNAS received a Polaroid camera at age eight and made inventive portraits of her pet schnoodle, Emily. By eighteen, she'd expanded her activities to include yoga, meditation, and college. She has since studied with several masterful yoga teachers, including Sofia Diaz, whose student she became in 2003. She holds an MFA from the Bennington Writing Seminars, and has written Internet-based articles on everything from firefighter training to nursing, plus several contemplative essays for *Yoga Journal*'s Conference Connection. She writes and teaches yoga in Colorado with her partner, who is a Zen monastery resident. She gets up really early.

JOHN FRIEND is the Founder of Anusara® yoga and is one of the most influential yoga teachers in the world. He was introduced to yoga in 1967, and began to practice and study at age thirteen. A yoga teacher for thirty-eight years, John has taught over 700 workshops in more than twenty-five countries. John is a visionary for blending a positive, life-affirming Tantric philosophy with Universal Principles of Alignment, and creating a heart-oriented global community. In thirteen years, Anusara yoga has grown to over 1200 teachers and 600,000 students in more than 100 countries. John is renowned for his charisma, knowledge, and accessibility. Connecting to the heart of each person, he ignites students to express the poses fully as a delightful dance of freedom. Above all, he sees everyone as a unique expression of the divine. Each practice with John is a path of awakening to our true nature and of celebrating the creative artistry of life through the body.

STEVE JACOBSON has studied and taught philosophy and yoga for many years. In philosophy, he is fascinated by epistemology in the British and American analytic tradition. In yoga he focuses on interrelations between body, mind, and breath. He also does simple wood working: his favorite tool is a DeWalt power drill.

JEFF LOGAN is the co-owner of Body and Soul Fitness and Yoga Center in Huntington, New York, which offers over 40 classes a week to this bustling Long Island Community. Jeff began his study and practice of yoga in 1982, and, leaving behind a twelve-year career as a bank executive, began teaching yoga in 1992. He is certified in the renowned Iyengar tradition and has studied with the Iyengars in Pune, India. Jeff has been interviewed frequently on the subject of yoga by various local and regional newspapers and has published yoga articles in magazines such as *American Association of Retired Persons, Runner's World*, and *Yoga Journal*.

PAUL ULHAS MACNEILL is professor and director of ethics teaching in the Yong Loo Lin School of Medicine, National University of Singapore. He previously taught ethics to medical students at the Universities of Sydney and New South Wales. He is a former president of the Australasian Bioethics Association and was Convener and President of the 7th World Congress of Bioethics held in Sydney in 2004. He is an active yoga practitioner, practicing principally with John Friend, Craig Sharp, and (now) various teachers in Singapore. He was a teacher of Siddha yoga meditation and Kyokushinkai karate.

KIERAN MCMANUS is a professional musician and IT consultant living in Maine. With a degree in French from Loyola College and a passion for exploring the world, Kieran has lived in France, Tanzania, Wyoming, and India. Most recently, he traveled with his 'cello around Nepal and India, recording music and trekking the Annapurna Circuit before finding an ashram in which to study yoga and meditation. His primary interest is music, and for the past twenty years Kieran has been writing, recording, and performing his spirited folk fusion of 'cello and guitar music. His most recent album, *Yellow Moon Over Portland*, can be heard on his website at www.kieranmcmanus.com.

NOTES ON CONTRIBUTORS

DEBRA MERSKIN watches her four-footed companions enact downward dog and cat stretches every day. She tries to emulate them and other animals in her yoga practice. Her scholarship addresses the symbolic representations of animals and humans in mass media. A recent article, 'Hearing voices: The promise of participatory action research for animals,' was written to extend her communication scholarship to applications with all beings. She lives in Eugene, Oregon where these kinds of ideas are considered normal. Her day job is as an associate professor in the School of Journalism and Communication at the University of Oregon.

JENNIFER MUNYER has had a deep respect for each person's unique journey in life since she witnessed and experienced the life-changing events of divorce. Her curiosity about life choices took her on a path of exploring psychology, health arts and sciences, religion, bodywork, embodiment, and, of course, yoga. Jen is the assistant director of programs for Phoenix Rising Yoga Therapy and lives in the great state of Vermont. She is ever grateful for the support of her partner and two incredible dogs.

J. NEIL OTTE was raised in Kansas, first by Methodists and later by members of the Kwan Um School of Zen. This early East–West education led to a lifelong fascination with the basic questions of philosophy, with an eye toward how cultural conversations can give us insight into the presuppositions of our own beliefs. His research touches on the history of materialism, posthumanism, the arts, and the relationship between conceptions of selfhood and ethical agency. He teaches at John Jay College in New York City and spends his mornings on a mountaintop in full lotus, facing east.

JULINNA OXLEY is a philosophy teacher at Coastal Carolina University. She discovered yoga on a trip to India, where she met the Dalai Lama, in summer 2001. She has practiced many different styles of yoga, but has maintained an Ashtanga yoga home practice for several years. Her book, *The Moral Dimensions of Empathy*, reflects her interest in emotions that are important in the yogic tradition. She lives in South Carolina with her husband Philip Whalen and her toddler Marigny, who loves yoga and has mastered 'downward pooping dog.'

BARBARA PURCELL is a New York City-based yoga instructor and writer covering such topics as urban holistic living, relaxation techniques, and results-oriented enlightenment. She started practicing yoga in 2000 as a way to combat the deleterious effects of Y2K, and began teaching several years later in an effort to prepare those around her for the anticipated apocalypse in 2012. (Don't worry – you've likely survived Y2K and quite possibly 2012, depending upon when you're reading this.) Barbara has been featured on a variety of TV and radio shows, most notably the *Tyra Banks Show*, helping couples with stress relief.

DAVID ROBLES is a Vinyasa yoga teacher with a lifelong interest in religion, philosophy, and mysticism. Along with his wonderfully talented wife, Adrea, he is the owner of Liberation Yoga & Wellness Center in Mahopac, NY. When he's not teaching people how to levitate, he enjoys studying Sanskrit with Swami Prabuddhananda Saraswati, reading voraciously, standing on his hands, tipping sacred cows, corrupting youth, and generally making a spiritual nuisance of himself.

HEATHER SALAZAR's interest in meditation, philosophy, and yoga started early. After becoming enmeshed in the frenzy of overdoing, she made it her mantra to *be* more and do less. She devoted her life to balance, openness, and appreciation of the wonders of life. Heather is enchanted by trees, sunshine, and animals of all kinds. She loves to hike and her favorite yoga pose is dancer. She is an assistant professor of philosophy at Western New England University where she teaches and writes about ethics and philosophy of mind. She also teaches mindfulness meditation and creates meditation art. Heather's current crowning achievement is getting her ethics class to chant 'om' six times (they loved it!).

ANDREW SHAFFER is the author of *Great Philosophers who Failed at Love*, a non-fiction book about the romantic lives of thirty-seven of the world's best-known philosophers. He is a regular contributor to *The Huffington Post*, as well as creative director of Order of St. Nick, the greeting card company whose irreverent cards have been featured on popular media outlets such as *The Colbert Report* and NPR. The first time Andrew attempted yoga at a local gym, he pulled a groin muscle and never returned. Visit him online at www.greatphilosophersbook.com.

ERIC SWAN earned his BA in psychology and MEd in guidance and counseling from Loyola College in Maryland. His interests in the Far East and meditation led him to pursue a Post-Master's Certificate in Spiritual and Existential Counseling at Johns Hopkins University, where he was introduced to Patañjali and yoga as a means for higher consciousness. It was not until Eric started practicing with his wife (and yoga teacher) Liz Swan, and Kitty Moore (of Sadhana West in Niwot, CO), that he developed a deeper appreciation for Hatha yoga. As an educator and counselor, he is interested in promoting yoga as a means for personal and social growth, relaxation, and health. He looks forward to practicing yoga with his son, who will undoubtedly have better flexibility than his dad. Eric continues to write and record original music, thanks to the support of his wife and his valued friend and fellow contributor to this volume, Kieran McManus. Long live Acoustic Oregon! Visit www.ericswan.org for more.

LIZ STILLWAGGON SWAN is delighted to have had the opportunity to produce a book about two of her favorite things in life: yoga and philosophy! Her seven-year yoga practice has been most strongly influenced by the Iyengar and Anusara traditions, but she is happy to explore new styles of yoga all the time. She had the pleasure of teaching a candlelight gentle yoga class in Kitty Moore's wonderful yoga studio in Niwot, CO (Sadhana West) and plans to return to teaching yoga now that her son Freeman is ready to do some yoga outside the womb!

ABBY THOMPSON has been practicing yoga since high school and teaching since 2008. Her experiences led her to pursue a graduate degree in somatic psychology. She recently relocated from New York City to San Francisco, and is still waiting for the jet lag to pass. She can't understand why her 'Yoga for Weary Time Travelers' DVD series hasn't sold well.